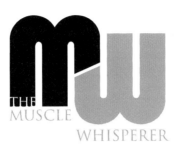

THE
MUSCLE
WHISPERER

DESPERATELY SEEKING A PAIN FREE SELF

RELIEVE PHYSICAL NECK, SHOULDER AND BACK PAIN
WITH A RETURN TO THE INNER SELF.

SOPHIA KUPSE

For more information please visit: **www.themusclewhisperer.co.uk**

PAINLESS PUBLISHING

ISBN-13: 978-1515033240

DEDICATION

This book would never have been possible without the endless stream of clients both in the UK and overseas, who have acknowledged and supported my work over the years. They are real heroes whose lives have helped so many and in exchange, they have suffered so much pain. Thank you for sharing your stories and being part of the process which allowed 'LT Therapy' to evolve.

CONTENTS

ACKNOWLEDGMENTS

FIONA KIRK NUTRITIONIST, AUTHOR & FRIEND – once again coming to my publishing rescue

MAX MORRIS MILKBAR CREATIVE – For putting book 2 together

DAVID CLARKE ROCK PR – My brilliant PR man

LAURA KUPSE 'CAULDRON OF MISCHIEF' – Thank you to my creative designer daughter Laura for all the body diagrams in Book 2 www.cauldronofmischief.co.uk & .com

MY FAMILY – For being good listeners

INTRODUCTION

After the success of my first book 'The Muscle Whisperer-The Keys To Unlocking Your Back Pain' I was inundated with requests from people all over the world, asking me to write more about the fascinating link between our physical pain and the mind. This in depth self help book, allows the reader to look at their own back pain from another perspective, to understand the way in which we converse with ourselves, can have a profound effect on our physical wellbeing. The additional information provided in this book covers why we feel back pain in the most common places such as neck, shoulders and lower back. It identifies what defines our physical pain and how we, if there are no contributory outside factors such as genetic disorders, accidents, and trauma, are solely responsible for its creation through our lifestyle choices.

If your muscles could talk, what would they say about you? Our muscles hold the key to our life's story. The body is like a timeline, in Eastern medicine the front of our body represents our present state and the back represents our past, our history. When I look at a person's back, it reads like a book and like a book, the human spine divides the pages; the left side of the body being male energy, Yang and the right side being female energy, Yin. I begin by using 'LT Therapy,' the technique I founded. It allows me to read each muscle bands pressure, by determining how supple the texture is under my fingertips. Both sides of the back must balance in order to bring flexibility, mobility and well being to the body. Based on the muscles location and tightness, I can feel from years of experience and intuition, any emotional or physical trauma held from as far back as childhood to the present day. By determining why these muscles are held in a state of shock, I can reset muscle memory, like reprogramming a computer, thus releasing the physical, as well as emotional pain held. It takes three key elements to do this, firstly, volcanic heat to transcend into the muscle and loosen any lactic acid held around the sensory nerves, discharging negative energy. All tightness held in the muscles correlates to negative memories which produce negative energy. Secondly, manipulation will unhook harmful negative attachments and allow me to identify the person, place or event connected to the client creating their physical or emotional pain. The client can respond verbally, confirming the events linked to that muscles timeframe and talk about it if they wish. Lastly, ice marble sweeps down into the muscle to restore positive energy and acts as a natural anti inflammatory, muscle memory is reset.

'LT Therapy' is like an extension of psychotherapy and physiotherapy, it is a two way treatment that helps the mind and body identify why we create our physical pain when all else fails. Every time we give a negative response to a situation, we hook the negative memory into the muscle. The muscles in the back, neck and shoulders are the main groups that take the impact, as they are our biggest muscle groups; if they are blocked then referral pain can be felt in the head, arms and legs. As the client speaks about their experience, they are releasing the memory verbally as I release it physically. When I reset muscle memory it is like I am removing an invisible fish hook from the muscle and the client unhooks the hook in their mind. When we are upset, stressed, angry, annoyed, emotionally compromised, we release adrenaline as our body prepares to activate the 'fight or flight' response. We hold ourselves physically stiff, our muscles are tense. We are preparing ourselves for battle, even if it is within ourselves. Over time, these continual mini battles, which are our stress responses to daily challenges, build and eventually, lead to physical pain we feel in the body. If we attach other known contributory factors to the blend, busy lifestyle, poor diet, and lack of exercise, is it any wonder we suffer so much.

I seem to spend most of the time in my clinic listening to my wonderful clients telling me how they have been down every western medicine route and still drawn a blank as to why they have the pain they do. If there hasn't been evidence of a fall, physical trauma, accident, genetic condition or intervention of an operation, then the doctors and specialists conclude its wear and tear. No matter how old my clients are and they range from 15 to 85, its wear and tear. Let's get one thing straight from the very beginning, the human body is a magnificent machine that can labour physically for a thousand hours, multi tasking strengthens our muscles working closely with our beautiful frame. According to Albert Einstein 90% of our brain sits idle, our brain is the human computer. Today's latest evidence states it is a myth that it only uses 10% to run all our twelve body systems, we actually use all of it in a continual process of learning. The human brain is one of the most powerful organs we have as it controls the functions of the body. It is sometimes referred to as a muscle of thinking as the brain actually tells our muscles what to do through the muscle memory process. The brain is the most important organ in the body because it controls all of the bodily functions as well as the other organs; therefore it has plenty to do and is constantly performing unconscious processes. Even when we sleep, most of the brain is active. The brain regulates everything from our heart rate and our senses to our dreams and emotions - so the brain is kept very busy. We use different parts of our brains in different ways when we do different tasks, so no part is unused. It is this understanding of the power of conscious and unconscious mind linking the brain that helps to regulate our emotions to that which creates our physical pain.

When you read through the following chapters you will begin to piece together how your brain, absorbs like a sponge, the language you use when speaking to yourself (and we all do), the way you think and your cognitive behaviour patterns from childhood, all contribute to physical pain. I want you by the end of this book to be able to not only understand this process, but actually be able to take control of it. You will be able to identify which parts of your back muscles store memories of key people and events in your life and how to go about releasing the tension held. As fast as you created your pain, you will be able to heal it. The power of the mind has no boundaries and the only limits, are the ones you create and place on it.

Most people come to my clinic looking for a miracle cure, a one stop treatment shop that after one session will restore their life back to how they would like it. Unfortunately, in today's world no one can perform such miracles or make such claims. I can reset muscle memory using 'LT therapy' and give you the tools to improve your life to make dramatic changes for the better, but no other human being is responsible for how you control your thoughts, what you eat and how much exercise you do. Yes they may help facilitate them, by knowing how to push your buttons, to trigger a negative response, but in the end, it is all down to you and the decisions you make. In order to help your physical pain improve you have to change the way you think, you have to break the habits and patterns that you have lived your life in and begin to form new ones, regardless of age. As we get older it is easier to stay set in our ways. By blaming others for the lack of who you are and what you have become and not achieved, is a result of a person living in their inner child. Over the forthcoming chapters you will learn and understand the importance of this and like a 'light bulb moment' start your journey of restoration of mind, body and spirit.

1

UNDERSTANDING OUR MIND

'If you want to win me over you'll deal with my mind and not my lips'
Dorothy Michaels From the movie 'Tootsie.'

Julie Andrews sang 'Let's start at the very beginning, a very good place to start' the song 'Do-Re-Mi' from the musical and movie 'The Sound of Music.' A film that became internationally loved by millions and adored by generations, why? This delightful story had a relatively unknown cast at the time, except for the lead actors, but regardless of any difficulties during the shooting of it, once the finishing touches had been made, it entered our history books as the most loved movie of all time.

What was it that made me, my family and my children, three different generations, all fall in love with it. Was it the songs, the music, the story, the scenery, the characters. Yes I can hear you shouting - all of it. The film based on the memoirs of Maria Von Trapp, set just before the Second World War in Austria, reflects the difficulties of a family without a mother and the relationship between their father the Captain and the governess. It blossoms into a love story and like all fairy tales, has a 'happy ever after' ending.

That's what every human being most of the time, seeks to achieve in their life, this ending of success and accolades. We are conditioned from childhood, whether at school, in story time, or at home via our parents or grandparents reading to us at bedtime and we, in turn read to our own children, the same 'happy ever after' stories. Planting the seed that all stories end this way and thus we concur that our life's journey should be the same. Our goals are usually set out by our ancestors a reflection of success is; the great job that comes after years of studying, the detached house that comes with the great pay cheque, the flash car that shows your peers you've made it, the loving partner that creates with you two perfect children, one girl and one boy, the endless annual luxury holidays to keep you all happy, but in reality it is far from this fairytale. The Disney corporation make billions creating the dream we all seek the' happy ever after.' But when such an ending does not occur in our life, we feel let down, disappointed, cheated that it never ever existed. Then who is to blame for this outcome. Humans like to hold someone responsible for failure, make them accountable for not delivering the 'happy ever after' who do you hold responsible for your 'not so happy ending.' Your parents, grandparents, partner, husband, wife, siblings, boss, friends, god- the list is endless and so personal as each of us develops our own blame list that is unique to us, to our story.

Eric Berne was a Canadian-born psychiatrist best known as the creator of transactional analysis and author of Games People Play. Transactional analysis (abbreviated to TA), is a theory in psychology that examines the interactions, or 'transactions', between a person and other people. The underlying principle is that humans are social creatures and that a person is a multi-faceted being that changes when in contact with another person in their world.   Berne suggests there are three "ego states" —the Parent-Adult-Child—which were largely shaped through childhood experiences. Unhealthy or difficult childhood experiences can lead to the Child and Parent ego states to develop deeper in the mind and build in adulthood.

I have used the basis of Berne's theory to show people how this 'ego state' which hosts all three, lives in both the conscious and subconscious mind and are key players in creating our physical pain. Now let's keep it simple, as understanding psychology can be a maze we lose ourselves in.

THE POWER OF THREE

Have you ever noticed that the number three is a dominant feature in our lives and the world. We use so many forms of it in numerical and written language to describe things, here's a few to think about;

The best of 3, 3 in 1, top 3, on the count of three, in religion the holy trinity, one in three, third time lucky, good luck but especially bad luck 'comes in three 'in sport they use the 'three second rule' a hat trick three successes on three consecutive occasions and so on. I'm sure you have a few of your own. Is this just a coincidence that has evolved over time or as man has developed so has the symbol three. Even we are made up after all of mind, body spirit and so the theory of being three people in one is no longer a mere fantasy, in psychology it truly exists and is what dominates our personality.

As I worked in my clinics with hundreds of people from across all walks of life, from different nationalities and cultures, I discovered that they all shared a common factor. Besides coming to me for help in resolving their back pain, pain being the obvious link, there was a more hidden, not so obvious reason. They all struggled with the lack of respect, value and love in their lives. The majority of people I treated were global success stories, multi millionaires, even celebrities in their own right, but they still felt a huge piece of their emotional jigsaw was missing and time was running out to find it. Where does this loss of value stem from, could it be varying or does it always starts from birth. This is a question I frequently asked myself over the years and finally concluded that regardless of how charmed a childhood a person had, there was always a deep pocket which was filled with unhappy memories and this was where the pain bug lived. Like most bugs, in order to grow, one must feed it and the more negative emotions we feed the bug that lives in our childhood pocket of 'lack 'the more it grows. We as humans need the power of '3' these key emotions essential to our survival, love, respect and value. Our search for these three vital components can make us or break us. If we succeed in finding all three throughout our lives we become balanced, satisfied, grounded, loving, kind, generous, gentle, humanitarians who give unconditionally. If we do not win these prizes, then we've lost the game of life, we lose ourselves and the price is poor mental health and reduced quality of physical ability. A stressed depressed person will emotionally eat and put on extreme weight or do the opposite, eat less, drink more and be extremely under weight. Finding the balance is the recipe for our salvation.

SALLY'S STORY

Sally a lovely client of mine built her battle with relationships and self worth all because of being rejected in her primary school years by her teacher. She was always a keen sports woman and wanted to join the football and rugby team, but was constantly told 'no girls allowed' only boys as they were all male dominated sports. Regardless of her showing great skill and potential, she was constantly denied the opportunity to play. She was well cared for by her parents, but the discipline at home and lack of tactility made her keep this rejection to herself. The frustration, rejection and the feeling of not being valued in childhood became part of her belief system and followed her throughout her life. When you do not resolve limiting beliefs such as this, you brand it in your memory and it becomes a habit. Every time your mind revisits it and Sally still does, she vividly remembers great details to the point of filling with tears. Her brain believes that the event is actually happening, it does not distinguish it is only a memory from the past. Due to Sally's real emotions she releases adrenaline and tears begin to form. She feeds her pocket of lack and it continues to grow. Sally wanted to end her back pain that had been with her since her late teens and endless visits to the physio and chiropractor over years had not resolved it. By resetting her muscle memory with my method I clearly identified the key areas that were blocked, what the cause was and who created it. Once identified, Sally could begin her journey of recovery. I gave her a guide to help her move forward by supporting her muscle memory and mind (see Chapter9) she would then return within 4 weeks in order for me to distinguish which areas, if any, she was re-blocking, then I would reset those again. I saw her 4 weeks later and amazingly her pain had virtually gone; only a slight tightness remained in her primary years which was the main area of concern. I reset her muscle memory again and emphasised the need for her now to move forward using the tools that I had given her, there was no looking back. Six weeks later Sally emailed me to say her pain had gone and even though she had days where she lost focus and slipped into a moment of feeling undervalued, which could trigger tension in her back, she quickly learned to feel the emotion and let it go. She was no longer adding to the pocket, she was no longer feeding her bug.

We create within ourselves many layers of different people that we meet over time. We absorb their mannerisms, we watch, we learn, we take what we like and what we don't like and voila! We have produced our personality. Over time we manufacture the adult we want the world to see us as, by expanding our knowledge, learning new skills and feasting on what success means to us, we do this to fit in, so we should be happy with the outcome, but we're not. This is because we develop a social front, and hide anything that doesn't appear 'normal' within ourselves, behind closed doors in order for society to accept us into the clan. The clan of belonging. We want them to see us as ordinary people, average, conventional, creatures of habit like them. We don't want our friends, neighbours, peers, to judge us or see us as any different or we would feel an outcast, an alien, as we need to be accepted and liked. But what is 'normal' these days.

I have to cast my net out and look way back to my own childhood when society truly made you feel the outcast from the clan and gave you a coat of 'not so many colours' like Joseph, but a coat of 'odd one out.' In 1968 aged 5, I started at the local Roman Catholic primary school. As my family were all Roman Catholics it made sense to be educated this way. I have very vivid memories of my earlier school years and the decade in secondary school that followed. Like most people, there was always some element of bullying going on and I was fortunate enough to bag some real gems. It was hard growing up with an unusual name 'Sophia Kolacs' named after Sophia Loren, Italian screen siren and sex goddess, I never quite filled her shoes, and topped with a Hungarian surname, was guaranteed to be the 'odd bod.' If people keep putting you in the 'your unusual' 'your different' category, well that's great in this millennium era, the more bizarre you are the better, but not back then. It was exactly what guaranteed you 'weirdo' status and if you just happened to have a Roman nose, unusual features and glasses, you got the 'abnormal' label. No matter how clever you were it was your name and looks that earned you the title. Your peers would go round sneering, gossiping, whispering and ignoring you. This continual behaviour pattern convinced you that they must be right and eventually you begin to believe their statement, that you were so different therefore did not belong in 'the clan' where all the 'normal' people lived. I remember standing in the primary school playground on a smoggy winter morning. It was freezing cold and I couldn't quite get my fingerless gloves on, so I had my hands in either side of my little fur lined anorak coat pockets. No one would play with me, I looked and felt so sad. I can still recall and feel those emotions so vividly today. I stood there looking at all the children playing, of which half of them just stared at me like I was from another planet, whilst the other half rejected me into their group. But I was from another planet because my name was like no other in the school. When the register was taken every morning, how I yearned for my name to be called out as Elisabeth, Susan or Ann, anything that fitted in because right now, I did not belong and my peers made me know it.

MUSCLE MEMORY

Rejection in the earlier years, whether at home or school is like a marker ingrained in the brain. It's filed in the subconscious mind under 'No Value.' This file can grow and has an excellent expansion chamber, so I can add many experiences of such rejection and believe it. The brain does not understand the difference between reality and fantasy, it does not know the past from the present, it lives on memory, so what you think it believes. How many times do you tell yourself one of the stories from this file. The 'no value' file, how many examples from your history, like me, can you recall. The more you keep on recalling, the more you experience the negative event all over again registering it in your physical body. It is proven that when we remember past events, we actually do not recall the original memory in its unique state, what we access is what we remember from the last time we recalled that memory. We actually add to the story and making it more colourful, more real in our mind. Just like in 'Chinese whispers' the more you retell it, the bigger the story grows. You don't realise that by doing this, you are creating physical pain in your body and affecting your cells and pre-disposed conditions to eventually come to the surface. This is done through muscle memory, our bodies advanced and complex network system of sensory nerves connecting communication links to the brain from under the muscles, allowing us to move without thinking. This same system allows our emotional responses, whether happy or sad, to travel down the same line. Most of the time we are in a state of negativity. Negative thoughts release adrenaline and cortisol. Unused adrenaline and cortisol leaves the body via our body's waste route, but residual amounts convert into lactic acid and get stored in the muscle groups. So if you're not continually running for a bus, exercising nonstop, then you are manufacturing these hormone responses in a sedentary state. The more stressed, angry, upset, annoyed, frustrated you are the more you build up these small layers of lactic acid. These layers construct in various muscle groups of the body until after time, they form trigger points known commonly as knots. Muscle memory not only independently works to move the body, but it continually records your thoughts, the chatter in your brain, happy thoughts generate the release of the happy hormones dopamine, serotonin, oxytocin that heal the body. Negative thoughts increase adrenaline and cortisol production storing lactic acid in the big muscle groups, the back being one of the largest muscle groups of the body. Hence my work grew from a need to understand why we suffer so much from neck, shoulder and back pain, when we as humans are built like machines. We are built to push our bodies to the limit and recover quickly, but it's the impact of stress and how it disconnects the balance of power within us that caused me to create the 'Langellotti Tri Therapy,' 'LT Therapy' as it is generally known.

THE FOUNDATIONS OF 'LT THERAPY'

When I treat a client with 'LT Therapy' to release acute and chronic muscular pain in the back, I incorporate elements of Yin Yang. In traditional Chinese medicine, illness is believed to be caused by an imbalance of yin and yang in the body. Even though it is the foundation of diagnosis and treatment in Chinese medicine, I only use a few key elements of Yin and Yang with 'LT Therapy.'

'LT Therapy' can be used on all parts of the body to release pain, but the torso is the mother ship of the body, housing the largest muscle groups. It is therefore the key area to release first, in order for the rest of the body to function normally. If a muscle is not working correctly in the back you can be guaranteed over time, the sensory nerves will become blocked in that area and referral pain in the head, arms or legs will be felt. I see many clients in my clinic with Rotator Cuff, Frozen Shoulder, Tennis Elbow, tingling sensations down the arms, Sciatica and they are on the increase. Yet again, western medicine dictates its wear and tear, which I agree to some extent, but the impact of our negative thoughts that block these areas, by tightening muscles groups and sensory nerves, is also a key contributor and has to be acknowledged at some stage. In order to release and treat these conditions, you need to start from the source. The original point where the energy blocked, that contributed to forming these conditions are all located in various muscles groups of the back.

The neck, shoulder and back muscles store lactic build up, formed from the release of adrenaline and cortisol, not just through our physical action, but also our negative thoughts, as negative thoughts become our worry, our stress. Lactic deposits build to form small or large knots; the size can vary depending on how long the area has been agitated physically or mentally. If mentally, it is the period of time you have been thinking about the problems or challenging events in your life. The knot will eventually put pressure on a sensory nerve and transmit a message of pain to the area of concern.

Eastern medicine reinforces this message of the need to balance both sides of the body or physical pain and disease will be unleashed if the status quo is not met. 'LT Therapy' applies this principle to the physical body and just as in reflexology of the feet, where the feet represents our complete mind and body systems, our neck, shoulders and back reflects our emotional belief system; including people, places and events that connect and affect our lives.

SICKNESS AND DISEASE

I experienced such illness in my mid 20's after helping my mother go through a very acrimonious divorce with my father.

After two long difficult years, I remember when it was all over, a week later I got up early for work, sat at the side of my bed and felt suddenly a great pain in my head as if it was about to explode. I truly believed it was a brain tumour, possibly formed after my head on collision accident on Christmas Eve, two years earlier. I collapsed on the floor hardly able to move. I requested a home visit from the locum doctor and sat on the floor waiting until he arrived. When he came an hour later, I was expecting him to admit me into hospital for a brain scan. Surprisingly, after doing all the usual body response checks, as well as looking into my eyes and ears, he put it down to a virus from M.E a condition I had never heard of, but he said it had been quite widespread and was well know as 'yuppie flu' the year was 1989 and M.E was in its infancy.

I had become a prisoner of this illness. A complete physical weakness dominated my body affecting my energy resources, respiratory patterns, cutting off my appetite and ability to concentrate on things for only a few minutes. I felt like a vegetable, just sat down on my sofa, useless to anyone. It took the best part of six months to build myself back up, using the same techniques as I did after my car accident in 1987. I applied visualisation and the self motivation methods I had learned to restore my wellbeing back then and it worked, yet again. I now know the trigger was the finalisation of my parent's divorce. The end of our family as a whole. It affected my foundations and hit it like a Tsunami wave. The after affects ripping through my inner child into adulthood. My childhood was far from perfect, in fact it was filled with verbal and physical abuse from my father, but regardless of that state, to the inner child, my little mini me had lost the parent combination and my dreams were shattered. I became the daughter of divorcees. For those who believe it does not affect a child, you are sadly mistaken. Whether you care to acknowledge it or not, it does affect your conscious or subconscious mind and will eventually surface. When I was a child growing up in such difficult circumstances, there was nothing I wished more, than for my parents to be divorced. I dreamed of living with my mother in more peaceful surroundings. Divorce for me as a teenager was the end of pain and the beginning of healing. Yet here I was now as an adult, battling an illness I did not ask for, but I did allow it in through the gates of my fragile mind. I remember as soon as the paperwork was over and the divorce was official, I walked out of the solicitor's office with my mother and before the ink was dry on the paper thought, now I can spend time focusing on my needs as I was mentally exhausted. I wanted time off to recover, but had no excuse to offer. Time out came in the form of my illness within seven days from me thinking it. Beware; such is the power of our beautiful mind.

You might say it was the strain of those two difficult years helping and supporting my mother that caused my illness to happen, but I doubt it. Looking back, I believe it was my inner child who was always searching to be part of a complete unit, it was the need to feel love and connection that caused it. I was sold as a child a belief of the perfect dream. In all the books I had read and there were many I escaped to, I lost myself in fiction to cover the cracks of a dysfunctional childhood. The stories I read, all had perfect families that I wanted to be part of, that was what my mini me believed and demanded. In reality, I as the adult knew better. We as individuals are always searching for the supportive parents, the love and acknowledgment we seem to need from them, but seldom get. I learnt that we can function perfectly well as a separated family, even better in most situations. So I will take my inner child by the hand and reassure her that this is not the end, but a new beginning that is far better than the old. When we can do this and truly believe in the three people we are parent, adult and inner child, we can all begin to heal both inside and out.

We live in a time where illnesses and disease have never been so out of control. These conditions are very real and can seriously debilitate a person to a virtual standstill, due to the chronic pain felt in the body, yet they are often disbelieved by family, friends and work colleagues. The exact cause of such 'new age' illnesses are still unknown, but they are strongly linked to stress related conditions such as anxiety and depression. We trigger these conditions and more, they are our minds cry for help, almost an automatic self harm button. When our needs are not being met from childhood onwards, then the feeling of rejection, lack of value, love and respect is activated. The three people we are need to be acknowledged and addressed. We need to familiarise ourselves with this state in order to start to understand who we really are inside. Only then can we start to stop inflicting ourselves with such physical pain.

2

ALL OF ME

'What's going on in that beautiful mind?... You're my end and my beginning...cause all of me loves all of you'

Lyrics & song by John Legend

Beautiful words from the song 'All of Me' by the modern day artist John Legend who wrote it for his future wife. But when I read the lyrics of this song, it fits so well with the 'who we are' inside. For copyright reasons I cannot reproduce all the words, but if you have a few minutes pop the artist and title of the song into You Tube and enjoy listening and reading every word. Even though it relates to two individual people, the song can be applied to the people within us. It cleverly tracks the journey of who we are within ourselves, the relationship between the adult and inner child. No matter what the original intention of the writer was behind the song, songs are interpreted by each listener in their own way. I found listening to this particular piece very profound and as I read each line on the screen I was saying those words to the 'little me' inside.

We all have a 'mini me'. Most of the time it's a regular joke as depicted in the Austin Power movies, but it's no joke when we start to ignore our 'mini me' because it starts to affect our well being.

DISCOVERING YOUR INNER CHILD

'The cry we hear from deep in our hearts comes from the wounded child within. Healing this inner child's pain will transform negative emotions and physical pain' Thich Nhat Hanh author of 'Understanding Our Mind.'

John Bradshaw a U.S. educator, pop psychology and self help movement leader, famously used "inner child" to point to unresolved childhood experiences and the lingering negative effects of childhood dysfunction. In this way "inner child" refers to the entire sum of mental-emotional memories stored in the sub-conscious from conception through pre-puberty.

In each of us, there is a young, suffering child. We have all had times of difficulty as children and many of us have experienced trauma, physical or mental abuse. To protect and defend ourselves against future suffering, we often try to forget those painful times. Every time we're in touch with the experience of suffering, we believe we can't bear it, and we push our feelings and memories deep down in our unconscious mind. We dare not face this child for fear of allowing our childhood traumas to surface, but yet they bleed into our lives.

But just because we may have ignored the child doesn't mean she or he doesn't exist. The inner child is always there, trying to get our attention. The child says, "I'm here. I'm here. You can't avoid me. Please accept me for who I am innocent, and playful.' The inner child is aged four to five, it is your gut feeling that you make your decisions on and if you listen and trust the inner child, it will never let you down. For the inner child is honest, trustworthy and never lies. Yet we try to shut it out. We want to end our suffering by sending the child to a deep place inside, ignoring its existence. But running away doesn't end our suffering; it only prolongs it.

Our inner child asks for care, love and respect, but we do the opposite. We do not face the child within us as we fear the suffering it may bring with it. The baggage of pain within us feels overwhelming. Even if we have time, we don't make time for ourselves. We try to keep ourselves constantly occupied— with other people's problems, watching television or movies, socialising, or using alcohol or drugs—because we don't want to experience that suffering all over again, we don't want to focus on us. Could this be one reason why our nation has become obese, due to emotional eating of processed high sugar and fatty foods, triggered by our inner child not being listened to or accepted for who it is?

The inner child is there, but we don't even acknowledge he/she is there. The inner child in us is a reality, but we can't see him/her and because of this inability to see, comes the ignorance of acknowledgement. This child has been severely wounded. He or she really needs us to recognise, allow and accept the inner child for who they are, but instead we turn the child away.

Allowing this ignorance affects our body and our consciousness. This ignorance stops us from seeing reality; it pushes us to do foolish things that make us suffer even more and hurt again the already-wounded child within us. It is this unawareness that creates our emotional battle within the conscious and subconscious mind.

The inner child is also in each cell of our body. There is no cell of our body that does not have that inner child in it. We don't have to look far into the past for that child. We only have to look deeply and we can be in touch with him/her. The suffering of that injured child is lying inside us right now in the present moment. If neglected and continually ignored, it will, like with any child who demands attention, start to kick off and this will result in illness or pain in the body. But just as the suffering is present in every cell of our body and creates our physical pain; it hides in the pockets of our muscle memory. We can use tools such as meditation and mindfulness to transcend into our mind and reach our inner child to say its ok you are safe, you are worth being here.

LISTEN

We must listen not only to others, but to the inner child inside us. That little child will try to constantly grab our attention from the depths of your consciousness and ask for your help. If you are mindful, you will hear his or her voice calling, at that moment, instead of paying attention to whatever is in front of you, go back and tenderly embrace the inner child. You can talk directly to the child lovingly saying, "In the past, I have ignored you, I am very sorry. I am going to embrace you." I am here for you. I will take good care of you. I know you suffer so much. I have been so busy. I have neglected you, I have not valued you.' If necessary, you have to cry together with that child. You have to talk to your child several times a day. Only then can healing take place. Embracing your inner child tenderly, you reassure him/her that you will never let him/her down again or leave him/her unattended. You begin the journey of valuing yourself as an individual in your own right.

If we look deeper, we can see that our inner child is not only us. Our inner child may represent several generations. Our mother may have suffered throughout her life. Our father may have suffered. Perhaps our parents weren't able to look after their inner child in themselves. We're embracing the inner child in us, we're embracing all the wounded children of our past generations, we are learning to break feeble habits that do not build strong foundations, we are no longer weakened by the limiting beliefs of our parent's teachings. They only passed on to us what was passed on to them. We inherited all their success as well as their disappointments. If they had any short comings in their life, you felt it. You almost took the blame for it, as if you were the cause of their losses in life, their failures. The lack of tactility, acknowledgment, reassurance, support, key mechanisms that a child needs for strong foundations are all missing, so when the child goes into adulthood this void of emotions starts to surface. We can do the same to our children, repeat the poor emotional process, the disconnection of cuddles and hugs or break the chain and give our children what we missed. If we can heal our inner child, we will not only liberate ourselves, but we will also help free whoever has hurt or abused us. The abuser may also have been the victim of abuse.

The people around us, our family and friends, may also have a severely wounded inner child inside. If we've managed to help ourselves, we can also help them. When we heal ourselves, our relationships with others become much easier. There is more peace and more love in us. Go back and take care of yourself. Your body needs you, your feelings need you, your inner child needs you. Your suffering needs you to acknowledge it. Daily practice of meditation, mindfulness and walking allows the mind to be free, think clear and thus leads to the body freeing itself from physical pain.

WHO CONTROLS WHAT IN THE MIND

The parent within us decides when the adult or inner child dominates the conversation in a nano second. The parent is like a referee and decides when to call each player into the decision making or conversation, depending on how our brain processes what we are doing at that very moment in time. Based on all our memories, experience and intuition we are either in our adult thinking mode or inner child mode. If the adult lives in the conscious mind and inner child in the subconscious mind, this relationship continues in the physical body.

When I ask people in my clinic at consultation point where they actually believe their muscular pain to be, they always point to the area of concern followed by a detailed explanation as to what physical cause they feel may have contributed to its creation. The usual reasons are; getting out of bed funny, picked up a box too quickly, turned awkwardly, spent too long at the computer, too many hours driving etc. Not one person ever, ever said it could be because I got so worked up over money, had an argument with my partner, fell out with my mum, upset the kids, was bullied by my boss, I just lost my dad etc. No one ever links physical pain to emotional or stress related situations, they may suspect it, but never acknowledge it; this is because as humans we need something tangible, something solid to blame. Emotions, feelings and stress can be felt but not physically touched. How can an emotion create a physical imbalance in the body? Easy, if every thought releases hormones to help us cope with whatever challenge we face, then the left over effects of hormones either heal or hinder our body. The more positive minded you are, the more you heal the mind and body, and the more negative you are the more you harm yourself. You've heard of people diagnosed with serious illnesses with little or no hope of a cure, but then because they changed their mindset from pessimistic to super focused and positive, they suddenly experienced a 'miraculous' recovery. It happened to me. Coincidence or not?

Just for a minute think of something that you can recall that makes you feel angry, upset or extremely sad. Watch how your breathing changes rapidly as the hormone adrenaline starts to enter the body preparing you with the 'ready to run' fight or flight feeling, but you're not running. How do your body and muscles feel - tense? Now start to calm down think of something that makes you feel happy and feel your breathing and heartbeat slow down, as the soothing hormones kick in like dopamine to heal you. One cancels the other out you may think and yes in theory it does, but in practice we never produce enough happy memories to counteract our painful ones. We are always out of balance, tipping towards the negative side of life, gravitating in the direction our peers, family and the media help us focus on. The brain cannot stop the negative chatter that goes on daily in our heads. It's a real conversation that happens and when people say they don't do it, they fear being ridiculed, because if you do talk to yourself, you must be mad. It's actually a very healthy and normal function of the brain to do this because we are made up of three people. As I said before, in psychology we are the parent to the adult and child within us. The adult dominates the conscious mind, whilst the child lives in the subconscious mind. So when we weigh things up, question things, make decisions we are always having a two way conversation with both sides of ourselves, the adult and the inner child and the parent is our referee.

OUR BACK, OUR MAP, OUR STORY

'LT Therapy' was developed to identify the links between physical pain and the negative thought process, recognising that thoughts can influence the state of how our body feels. 'LT Therapy' allows me to reset muscle memory, helps recognise the quality of the relationship we have with our adult side and inner child and how they influence our well being. A poor relationship with yourself can reflect in the form of depression, emotional eating, alcohol or drug abuse, weight issues, poor self esteem. A good relationship with yourself can result in success, feeling secure, loving the way you look and feel, helping others, eating healthy. Explaining this to a client can help them see a way forward in dealing with their state of pain or ill health, when western routes have failed. Making them understand how their negative mindset and limiting beliefs, control their reaction to things in their life, could eventually have a profound effect on their health, instantly or much later.

Our back carries our life story and through 'LT Therapy' I read the back like a map that has many hidden locations concealing pain. The only prize I discover behind each knot, is the reason why a person's pain was created and how it now relates to their life. The back is like your history book, it covers your past from childhood to the present day. Your spine is the divider, binding both the left side, male energy and right side, female energy together. Eastern medicine talks about balancing both these sides for total well being. When they become unbalanced, physical pain develops; pressure builds on top of the sensory nerves under the muscles, in the form of lactic knots. When the pressure is overwhelming, it sends a signal to the brain and suddenly, you start to rub your neck, shoulder or lower back, where you feel the pain, not knowing why. Each muscle group in the back relates to people, places and events, it is a time line linked to your life. Using a combination of several disciplines taken from extensive knowledge and experience, working in the field of Holistic medicine over 25 years and intuition, I explain to the client how their neck, shoulder and back pain came about, relating each area on the back to specific life pressures. It is a very insightful treatment and 80% of people find it a cathartic journey, a huge emotional release. Every person I see has a story unique to them, there may be similarities form person to person, but no two cases are alike, just as no two backs or their related pains are the same. I feel honoured that they have chosen me as part of their healing journey, to facilitate their well being. Each client is a radiant star in their own right, but they don't acknowledge it, after years of being told differently. They are all beautiful individuals, as we all are, fighting to stay in the game of life, battling to survive whatever it throws at us. If we are to win this game, do not play just to survive, play like a natural born leader, believe in both you and your inner child, unleash the super hero in you. I come across so many incredible stories testing human endurance, Traudi was no exception.

TRAUDI'S STORY

Traudi Schiller was an amazing lady I met at one of the health festivals I attended in York in the spring of 2015. I am always careful not to judge people when they present themselves to me. Society always pre-judges people, but nobody is who they seem, regardless of what they show up front. She had a delightful German accent which was almost bursting with effervescent fizz and filled with warmth. I find the German language difficult and harsh to master, so was surprised at how she made it sound so creamy and smooth, like milk chocolate melting in your mouth. Traudi had a way of making you feel at ease, as you were drawn into her healing aura. When she came to my clinic in West

Yorkshire, she presented me with her physical problems, one being deep pain in the left shoulder and a limiting ability to turn her neck. It had almost ceased full movement and she could only turn her head left to right by 30%, this was her gift from from an almost near fatal car accident 25 years earlier. These extreme physical symptoms gave her referral pain in the chest wall and into her shoulders, but I knew there was more of a story behind her physical pain.

She lay covered on my sports couch; face down with her neck, shoulders and back facing me. I only expose the part of the back I am working on in order to keep the other muscles comfortable and warm. As I began to apply the oils and pressure, I told Traudi what each area that was blocked in her back muscles related to and with a great sigh of relief, as if someone had finally supported her life, she said 'well that's no surprise.' Her left shoulder had started with Rotator Cuff problems as a by product of her neck issue, her sternocleidomastoid muscle, had lost most of its mobility. I pinpointed specific areas that held male energy that were severely blocked and related to a past husband, partners, her father and guardian. They were all negative influences in her life since childhood. As I went on to unravel more details, Traudi joined in. I previously explained to her that 'LT Therapy' is a two way treatment, an extension of physiotherapy and psychotherapy, if she wished to discuss my finding at the time of treatment; she could and would experience a deeper physical release in the muscles. As I physically released the trauma, she released it verbally and her muscle memory was reset using volcanic heat, ice marble and manipulation.

Traudi told me of her life in Germany, as a young child of 5, she lost both parents in the concentration camps. She went to live with her grandmother, her mother's sister and her husband who became her guardians. Her grandmother was her ally, who she loved dearly and taught her that no matter what life gave you, you had to give back. Her stepfather was cruel and starved her, he disliked girls and hoped she would starve to death, but against all odds she survived. She met and fell in love with an English businessman and soon fell pregnant. They decided to get married. Unfortunately, she lost her baby boy who was born in Berlin on 5th October 1965. They decided to move to England for a fresh start and she arrived Christmas 1965. She was young and innocent with no knowledge of the English language but she believed she would live out her new life in much happiness, would her fairytale come true.

Her husband turned out to be a bully, verbally abusive, her mother-in-law was the same. She endured over 40 years of marriage at the hands of her abuser, she had a further nine children and lost a daughter aged two months just before Christmas 1974. She learned to survive the loss of her babies and miscarriages as well as bring up the eight surviving children on her own. Her husband was an alcoholic and gambler so she couldn't rely on him to provide for the family. Education was extremely important to her; she felt it held the key to her freedom. In any spare moment she had, she studied lots of subject, passed her driving test, became fluent in English and in 1996 graduated as a teacher. Her husband continually called her a stupid woman, with a stupid silly accent. He belittled her because of the failure he felt inside him, as he tortured himself with alcohol and debts, he was dragging her down with him. Stress and worry continued to chase her throughout her life as she battled health problems. She instilled only positive values into her eight children who are today all thriving adults' leading successful lives. Now aged 72, Traudi is grateful to have survived kidney cancer in 2012 and still continues to live her life to the fullest capacity, doing kind deeds for others as she feels she still has a lot of love to give. She continues to work full time as a support worker, caring for less fortunate people in difficult circumstances and is a busy grandma to her delightful grandchildren.

Traudi's story is to be published, the book will be called 'The Girl who Survived Hitler's Third Reich.' She says of my work

'I have been so very glad I have been guided to meet you. I can now benefit from your amazing healing gift. I think you are fantastic, a natural healer who has done wonders for people all over the world. I already know after one treatment I feel much better in my mind and body, after suffering many years of pain, anguish and turmoil in my personal life. I have spent my life trying to improve and heal myself to overcome my anxieties. What attracted me to your work was the connection you make between physical pain and the mind. I know how powerful the mind is and what you tell it, it believes. I know the difficulties in my life created my health problems; you have now helped me confirm my thoughts on it. Thank you for developing 'LT Therapy' and restoring my wellbeing. I now have 80% improvement in my neck and shoulders, I am almost pain free. Looking forward to seeing you for my follow up appointment.'

No matter how painful our journey in life is and the challenges we have to face, if we learn to love the child within us, no matter how many times people put you down, you will always win. Traudi kept on believing in herself no matter how many times her husband put her down, but she never acknowledged her inner child. As I said before, it is the ignorance of not knowing your inner child is within you, that causes your physical battles. Learn to love all of you as in the words of John Legend, 'Cause I give you all of me and you give me all of you and all of me loves all of you.'

3

THE TREE OF LIFE

'Till we find our place on the path unwinding in the Circle of Life'
From 'The Lion King' Lyrics by Elton John

In botany a tree is a perennial plant with a trunk supporting branches and leaves. Trees tend to be long-lived, some reaching several thousand years old. Trees have been in existence on the Earth for 370 million years. They include a variety of plant species that have independently evolved a woody trunk and branches as a way to tower above other plants to compete for sunlight.

A tree typically has many secondary branches supported clear of the ground by the trunk. This trunk typically contains woody tissue for strength, and vascular tissue to carry materials from one part of the tree to another. For most trees it is surrounded by a layer of bark which serves as a protective barrier. Below the ground, the roots branch and spread out widely; they serve to anchor the tree and extract moisture and nutrients from the soil. Above ground, the branches divide into smaller branches and shoots. The shoots typically bear leaves, which capture light energy and convert it into sugars by photosynthesis, providing the food for the tree's growth and development. Trees play a significant role in reducing erosion and moderating the climate. Trees and forests provide a habitat for many species of animals and plants. Trees provide shade and shelter, timber for construction, fuel for cooking and heating, and fruit for food as well as having many other uses.

Humans are similar to trees, with the exception that we don't live on for several thousand years and glad not to. We have a trunk and our branches are our head, arms and legs. Our woody tissue that gives us strength is our muscles and the vascular tissue that carries material around our body is our circulatory system. Our layer of bark that acts as a protective barrier is our skin. Our smaller branches and shoots are our blood vessels, respiratory and regulating system, our eyes capture light and mouth aids absorption of nutrients. Our roots located at the base of the lower back, serve to anchor our childhood memories and belief system. We as humans are like trees, and play a significant role in the circle of life on this planet, providing food shelter for our loved ones and working towards helping climate change. **Diagram 1a** in this chapter shows the human back and our own tree of life layered on top.

The tree of life represents the emotional pathway in our body. By understanding where in our muscle groups, we store our pain, we can begin to be aware of what our pain can mirror. Suddenly, not all muscular pain falls into the 'wear and tear' category. Suddenly, we can start to take control and appreciate it could be due to our negative feelings. Our neck, shoulder and back muscles keep a daily record, like a register of how upset, angry, resentful, rejected, undervalued and unappreciated you feel. The tighter our muscles get, the more our pain impacts the muscles, causing restrictions in flexibility and mobility. Our body uses pain to tell us that something is not right. It allows you to push yourself so far and then, something's going to give and your health will be compromised. Then it's time to investigate the cause, in order to restore balance.

Tree Of Life

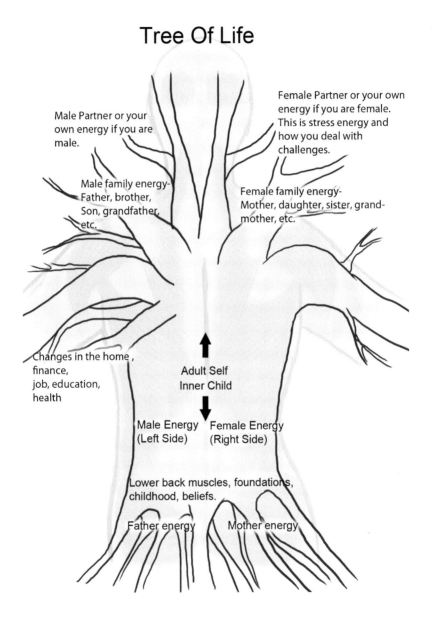

Male Partner or your own energy if you are male.

Female Partner or your own energy if you are female. This is stress energy and how you deal with challenges.

Male family energy-
Father, brother,
Son, grandfather,
etc.

Female family energy-
Mother, daughter, sister, grandmother, etc.

Changes in the home ,
finance,
job, education,
health

Adult Self
Inner Child

Male Energy
(Left Side)

Female Energy
(Right Side)

Lower back muscles, foundations,
childhood, beliefs.

Father energy

Mother energy

HOW DID THE TREE OF LIFE DEVELOP

By combining and applying the philosophies of psychology, eastern medicine and a vast amount of experience working with thousands of clients over the years, my method evolved. Energy work never fails to amaze me with the real results it delivers and working intuitively, allows a greater understanding to grow. The seed was planted and like an artist, with a vision, the tree of life grew. It was tested over 15 years before I really allowed myself to believe the remarkable results I attained. They were consistently positive and life changing. Receiving hundreds of testimonials from people saying how, after one treatment, they felt free to make decisions they feared to make before. They felt ready to let go of difficult relationships, changes in location and jobs. They coped better at accepting loss; they recovered from panic attacks and anxiety, but most of all, their pain had gone. I learned to never doubt myself and what I truly believed in, I've made my therapy my life's passion. I learned that your back, that represents your life story, never lies. No matter how the person presents them self to me, eventually their real story comes out. Some people mask their emotional pain by convincing themselves that their physical pain is all down to physical exertion, but no one lives a perfect life and the impact of lost feelings are very evident in their back.

Fear stops people moving forward, making the right decision, allowing them therapy. On occasion when people make appointments and are so keen to attend their first treatment with me, suddenly they genuinely fall ill, 24 hours before attending or less. I get a call saying how they've been struck down with gastric symptoms, or been sick all night or broke out in a temperature. It's their self sabotage system kicking in, the realisation that someone might be able to put a stop to all the years of physical pain, the inner childs conditioning reminds them that they are not worth it.

SAY HELLO TO YOUR 'MINI ME'

In March 2015 the NHS Choice magazine published an article based on a new study that found lower back pain to be among the top 10 health complaints in the world. Lower back pain may now be the leading cause of disability worldwide. It affects 1 in 10 people and is becoming more common with increasing age. The results of this research – which used data from a large study undertaken in 2010 on the global burden of disease – are likely to be reliable, and its findings will be of concern to health officials. Lower back pain can be acute or chronic. Though several risk factors have been identified such as occupational posture, depressive moods, obesity, body height or age, the causes of the onset of low back remain obscure and diagnosis difficult to make.

Lower back pain affects children to the elderly. In the UK lower back pain was identified as the most common cause of disability in young adults with more than 100 million work days lost each year. Many cases of back pain have no known cause. The study does a good job at highlighting a common, but often overlooked condition. Lower back pain is not usually linked to any serious disease, but can be debilitating and emotionally distressing.

If the Western world is struggling to find a reason as to why lower back pain is on the increase, with growing data to support its findings, then you have to seek your own resolution to deal with yours. Back pain is on the increase, especially lower back pain. The increases worldwide are a silent epidemic. Is it any surprise that our lower back, which symbolises our foundations, the roots of our beliefs deeply planted in the base of our back and controlled by our inner child, are so painful. When we silence the child within us, lower back pain occurs. We bury our inner child here and ignore it, is it any wonder we get such ongoing problems. The saying 'children should be seen not heard' comes to mind, how many people grew up with this message instilled in them. The older we get, we seem to encounter longer periods of discomfort in the lower back. We become more child like with age, our inner child is demanding relaxation, fun, laughter, joy, but instead we offer it the opposite. Time is passing us by so quickly, that we soon learn the importance of using it wisely; it's our body's natural way of making light of things, learning to play, have fun and brighten the days that have become so dark.

When I was in my early 20's and contemplated on starting a family I always thought the older you got, the less you would worry. Things would get easier. I know that belief is no longer true, my own mother now 80 and I, in my early 50's have become nonstop worriers. I help resolve my worry with daily meditation which alleviates any stress I feel, but mother finds it difficult breaking her lifelong conditioning. My clients from all ages, in their late teens and especially those from their mid 40's onwards, become anxious and apprehensive at most things in life. Is this because we live in a faster paced world compared to the 1950's when stores were closed on Sunday and it was seen as a family day. Strolls in the park, picnics, people made time for people, did we suffer the same amount of back pain then, as we do now?

HAVE YOU HEARD THE NEWS

If your focus is on negative things, you will become the result of it. You create the illusion of 'I can cope very well thank you' 'I don't need anyone's help' but really you are struggling inside. We are becoming a nation conditioned by pessimistic press reports, the failing NHS, the downfall of the economy and that no one ever retires, as there isn't enough in the pension pot. Is it any wonder we suffer so much back pain. How long do you spend watching the news every day? Probably longer than you think. You have it on the radio when you are eating your breakfast and getting ready for work. You have it on in the car, you read your news apps on the mobile phone or ipad, you can access it on your computer, you watch the evening news when you get home, you pick up a newspaper and it's there again. 99% of the news is all based on depressing subjects. I understand the importance of keeping up to date with the progress of the local and overseas news, but when it saturates our senses then it starts to alter our state. You follow this up with soaps such as Eastenders, Emmerdale, Hollyoaks, Home & Away which are again 80% drama based stories that are supposed to parallel and mimic our lives. Can you see the longer you absorb yourself in these messages your body will soak it up like a sponge, the more you train your brain to feel you need it, the more you will search for it like an addiction. I am all in favour of supporting media and the press, when you read informative, helpful pieces on health, beauty, food or lifestyle articles, but you have to learn to control what you watch. After 4 hours of negative TV per day, you listen to negative people at work, your boss has a go at you and your family are needing your support. You listen to their problems, you try and help them and everyone drains you. By the end of the day you are feeling worn down. You become stressed; anxious, overwhelmed and back pain sets in.

TIM'S STORY

Tim had worked with me in my early days, after leaving school to join the Civil service. I escaped eventually and developed my own practice over 20 years ago, but Tim had 32 years of loyal service behind him, when he contacted me for a treatment of LT therapy. Tim as I recalled, was a very chilled out man, took everything in his stride and was well known for his relaxed disposition, so I was really looking forward to catching up with a past colleague who worked at a sublimely relaxed pace, but always got the job done. Visually Tim had not changed much, he had looked after himself physically, but his mental state was another story. He had a wonderful home life, but things in the office had changed dramatically over the years. New procedures came in after a takeover and suddenly Tim was thrown into a world of intense targets, updated performance procedures, daily meetings, the list of changes were endless. The changes had come about gradually over the last five years, but the past 18 months were particularly intense. In that period of time, Tim's world at home took a huge hit, when his mother sadly passed away unexpectedly. The man, who was so chilled internally, was now in a tail spin, trying to keep it together and he did, but just. As he focused on hitting his new targets, he buried his grieve in paperwork, he didn't want to lose his job as well.

Tim's shoulders and neck were tight as a rock, so solid that he was experiencing referral pains in the chest and tingling in the arms. He also complained of chronic lower back pain particularly on the lower right side above the glute muscle. When clients see me for the first time, all I will ask for is their medical information, anything related to emotional and lifestyle changes, has to be discussed during the treatment. At the consultation he did not tell me anything about work and home, as usual Tim put the brave face of 'I can cope' on and 'my emotional upset has nothing to do with my physical pain' or has it?

When he lay on the sports couch I began to explain that his back represented his past, it held all emotional as well as physical trauma. The consultation had confirmed that he had suffered no physical trauma, so the pain was a build up of the changes at work and the loss of his mother. This I established by clarifying the key areas he felt were blocked, related to these events in his life. Top right shoulder lower neck was where a huge knot sat, this was his mother's energy in his adult life. Lower back right side was his mother's energy in his childhood years. The inner child was grieving for the loss of his mother whilst the adult was struggling to come to terms with the loss as well. The two parts connected as I knew they would, I worked to release the tightness and reset muscle memory to restore mobility to the treated area. I removed the physical memory of pain held in the muscle and left the original memory in the mind intact. I moved on to his left side, which represented work changes and bereavement. It was stored in the mid left back in the trapezius muscle band.

There were five tight knots the size of mini tangerines. As I worked on this area, explaining what they represented, he was amazed that I could identify all those personal details just by feeling his muscles. He then began to tell me about how work had changed beyond recognition, that he could keep up with the job, but the targets were pushing people to the limit. It had started to make his work colleagues and team members very negative, everybody was accountable for every minute of the day, they were all feeling the pressure. Tim never liked to be around pessimistic people and their attitude was now rubbing off on him. He was feeling depressed and began absorbing himself watching the news at least six times a day. His wife had pointed this out, that the only thing he watched was various news programmes nothing else. He went to work and soaked up other people's negativity. He understood now why he felt so much pain in his neck shoulders and lower back, as it did connect to all the issues in his life. By the time the treatment ended he couldn't believe the flexibility had returned so fast. For homecare, I recommended he changed what he watched. Limit the news to once a day and when he got home after work, watch comedy shows and comedians as well as funny films he used to love. This would re-engage his mind, release healing endorphins and restore a state of well being. He also had to focus what his job gave him, a salary to fund not only his lifestyle here, but his second residence in Spain, which would eventually be his retirement home. When I saw Tim a few weeks later for his review it was like seeing the old Tim again, a happier relaxed man, who ensured he made those key changes. He felt mentally more focused, slept better and 90% of his pain had gone. It was his mother's energy in the lower back that was still present, not as tight, but still there. I told him your inner child is aged 5 and no 5 year old wants to lose their mother. No matter how old you are as the adult, your inner child will never age. He had to work on his grief and we put things in place for him to support the inner child.

There are many people that go through what Tim has experienced every day, unhappy with their job, losing a loved one, dealing with difficult work colleagues, but you have to focus on the way forward, you have to change your minds response to the situation, or you will continue to struggle daily with those difficulties and they will grow bigger. By Tim understanding that he had to work with his inner child to resolve his lower back pain, he changed his focus and acknowledged his grief. He reassured his 'mini me' and made a good recovery.

WHAT A CHILD NEEDS

Why look at what a child needs and their values, when you are now all grown up? To understand ourselves and the inner child, we need to look at what are the optimum conditions to bring out the best in any child. Value and beliefs are learned in our primary years, strong beginnings are the core to a happy, balanced adult. When we miss elements from this process the child will suffer, we eventually suffer.

As we become adults our own values and beliefs have a critical impact on our self esteem, the way we make decisions, design programs and conduct ourselves. It is important to be clear about our personal values and beliefs and those shared as a group when working with others, making decisions that impact on others or undergoing changes. When an individual's, values and beliefs are challenged by others, we are asked to justify or account for our behaviour or when there is conflict about someone else's behaviour. In an ideal world a child needs;

- To feel secure, supported and valued in a cooperative and collaborative learning environment both at home and school.
- Optimal learning occurs when learning experiences cater to individual learning styles developmentally appropriate and authentically child-centred
- Confidence, competence and a positive self-identity come from valuing and supporting a childs diverse knowledge, skills and cultural understandings.

- Children learn best in environments that are responsive to their needs and strengths that allow them to feel safe, secure and nurtured.
- Play is an essential method of learning for young children that optimises the use of natural curiosity and enquiry, it is important to ensure play is made daily.
- Effective learning for children promotes the use of all their senses

How many of these processes did you have in your childhood? How many were missing? I am not writing this piece to point out your weaknesses, make you feel less than you should or criticise the way in which you were brought up. On the contrary, I want to heal your inner child and show you that it is never too late to introduce daily activities that build your values and self belief in you. In chapter 9 I give you a guide on how to do this and establish new ways which may help improve any physical back pain you suffer from.

We need to learn that it is never too late to acknowledge the inner child, your 'mini me.'

So many people tell me how well their parents brought them up, but the only thing they missed was a cuddle from mum or dad or both. The reassurance that everything would be alright, the praise for doing well instead of you can do better, the constant push. Depending on where you were in the pecking order dictated your fate. If you were the eldest, you felt responsibility was given to you at birth. How many people who were first born were made to look after their younger siblings, take a Saturday job or paper round, do their best at school always, there was always greater expectations on the first born. If it was a boy he seemed to be more loved, more respected than a girl or did that change with the decades. If you were the middle child (as I was) you were the doer, the helper, the giver, if you had an older sister you wore her hand me down's if you had an older brother you were lucky. I had the latter. If you were the youngest were you the fairest child of all. Were you told you were the favourite, the baby of the family, the special one; did you get away with more or less? This all affects our core beliefs, the order of our birth, the relationship we have with our siblings. The way we then viewed our parents and how we view them now, whether they are still with us or not. Do we pass judgement on family, are we drawn into their dramas, do we get caught up in the firing line of division of family property, do we still feel the prejudice of favouritism. You see now, why we must revisit our history not to dwell on it, as we cannot change the past and I am not expecting you to change your personality either. We revisit to access what cognitive values and behaviour patterns were missing in our childhood, then we move forward and create what our needs are now. We do not hold our self back with limiting beliefs established from our history. Remember these are your beliefs taken from the 'lack' file. We make these changes 'till we find our place on the path unwinding and join in the Circle of Life.'

4

HOW TO SELF DIAGNOSE YOUR BACK MUSCLES & NATURAL PAIN SOLUTIONS

'Getting to know you getting to know all about you'
From 'The King & I'

You have learned so far about the power of the mind and how your emotional response to life, can have a profound effect on your physical wellbeing. Your muscles hold so much encrypted historical information about how you emotionally react to people, places and events, it's time now to re-evaluate. If the way we react continues to serve us or by making a few constructive changes, we can introduce more balance, reduce pain and increase our wellbeing to a higher level.

Most of us understand the benefits of massage and how it makes us feel really good when our muscles are tight, tired, and sore. Even though we know this, many of us struggle to allow ourselves an opportunity to have a treatment. We make endless excuses of no time, no money, it always goes back to feeling the same, but new studies have now reinforced the importance of massage. Science tells us the reasons why and how massage not only feels good, but can actually help heal inflamed and damaged muscles. According to research conducted at McMaster University Ontario, Canada, massage therapy triggers sensors in the body to send out inflammation-reducing signals. The researchers believe the stretching of the muscle is what prompts the signal and encourages the healing process. In Chapter 9, I cover the importance of daily stretching and especially about the benefits of using a foam roller. Scientists believe massage could be a good alternative to pain medication for people as well as athletes looking to heal damaged muscles. In addition, because massage is causing an anti-inflammatory response, scientists are now also considering it as a way to help people suffering from arthritis, muscular dystrophy, and other chronic inflammatory diseases. But we need to look at the 'bigger' picture in order to resolve our pain.

EMOTIONAL ENERGY

If we look at our back and see how and where emotional energy forms, where people, places and events that create our world live, it would be like **diagram 2b and 3c.** It shows the location of the parent, inner child and adult, in the physical body and the areas they control. Remembering that the back represents our history and the front of our body represents our present time line. The influence of the adult and inner child's energy is also reflected in the front of the body. Let's look at where and what they connect with.

Energy and your partner

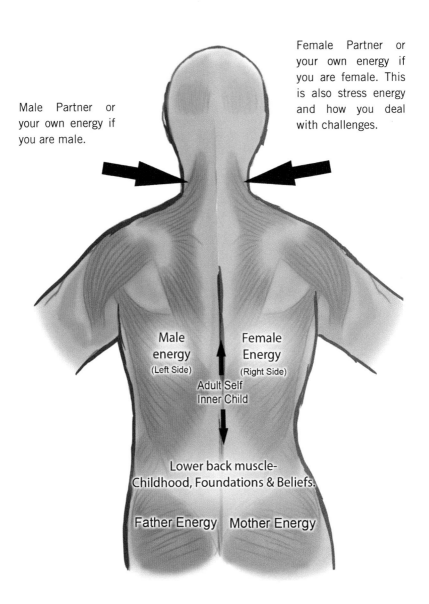

Female Partner or your own energy if you are female. This is also stress energy and how you deal with challenges.

Male Partner or your own energy if you are male.

Male energy
(Left Side)

Female Energy
(Right Side)

Adult Self
Inner Child

Lower back muscle–
Childhood, Foundations & Beliefs.

Father Energy   Mother Energy

Front of Body

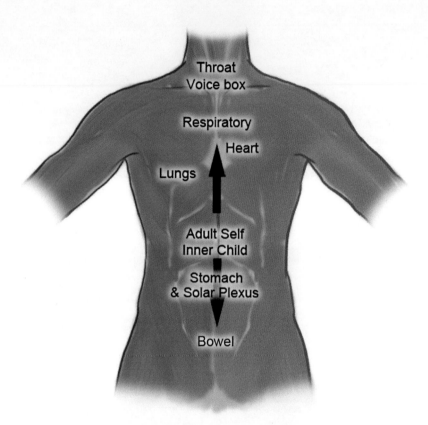

Our inner child influences the following parts of the back and front of the body;

Back of Body -The Lower to Mid Area

The lower back is the foundations of childhood. It is where our beliefs are firmly rooted. These are the beliefs we learned from the age of 3 to 8 from the beliefs of our parents or whoever brought you up. If you press your finger into the central part of the lower back, either side of the spine, you will come across two small indentations. There are either side of the sacrum. The right side is female energy, the left is male, so if you are female, the right indentation represents your birth point and the left side corresponds to the male birth point. From this position travelling up the middle of your back where the lattisimus dorsi muscle lays near the spine, is your primary and secondary years, these are 0-10 years old, 10-20 years old. If you are female you will be focusing on the right lower to mid back if you are male it will be the same, but on the left side of your back. Any discomfort pain or tightness in this area represents difficulties in your childhood, puberty and late teens till you are 20. Your Father's energy is located on the lower left side of the back, on the top of the gluteus maximus muscle (top of your left bottom cheek) and Mother's energy is on the lower right side of the back, on the top of the right gluteus maximus muscle. When you press on these areas as the diagram shows, you will feel how tender, tight or soft they feel, which represents your relationship with them in your childhood.

Front of Body -The Mid to Lower Area

The inner child controls the solar plexus which is the third chakra. The Solar Plexus Chakra, represents our ability to be confident and in control of our lives. It is located in the base of the stomach. The inner child also governs the stomach, bowels, appendix and all our internal organs in that region. Is it any wonder so many of us suffer with various ailments in these parts. Many times there is no explanation for the trigger of stomach acid, gastric problems, bowel issues such as IBS, colitis, food intolerances, food addictions, bulimia and anorexia. Keep a diary of days when you are emotionally more compromised and see how long it takes your body to react to the change. Problems in these areas are strongly linked to difficulties in childhood.

Our adult side influences the following parts of the back and front of the body;

Back of Body - Mid to Upper Area

The adult controls the muscles of the mid to upper back towards and including the shoulders and neck. I will discuss the shoulders and neck separately, I am focusing mainly on your trapezius muscle which dominates from the top of your shoulder, includes your shoulder blade and travels to half way down your back in a kite shape. Remember, the focus is on muscle not bone. The right side which is female energy Yin, is where we find females in our extended family like, aunty, niece, cousin, stepsister, stepmother, mother-in-law, sister-in-law. Our female friends are also located here as well as professional female work colleagues. It is also where affairs for both male or female, regardless of who caused it would be found. It is my job to determine during treatment who is causing emotional stress, if any or all. If you feel any discomfort or intense pain in this area, you have to focus on which female member/s of your family, work colleague/boss or friend caused you undue upset to produce such pain now or in the past. They may have let you down or you may be worrying about their health, wellbeing or you may be grieving for their loss. Again, if it relates to extended male members of the family, work colleagues or friends this would be in the same place, but on the left side of the back where all male energy is found.

Front of Body - Mid to Upper Area

The adult controls on the front of the body, from the mid section where the liver, heart, chest, respiratory, lungs are found to the upper area which includes the throat, voice box, swallowing reflux, trachea. Any issues with panic attacks, palpitations, AF, anxiety, chest infections, asthma, sore throats and thyroid issues are triggered by the negative emotions from the adult mind, which can also be linked to our core beliefs.

Shoulders & Neck

This is our crowning glory of hurt, where most of us manifest the majority of our pains. It will come as no surprise to learn that our nearest and dearest, those we hold so close to our hearts, give us our biggest aches. Once again, you'll be fed up of my constant reminders, but they are necessary and as W. Clement Stone businessman, philanthropist, new thought self help author says of repetition, 'you affect your subconscious mind by verbal repetition.' That is one of the aims of the book, by slowly repeating the message, albeit it presented in different ways in each chapter, you eventually will understand the need to acknowledge the inner child and bring more balance of male and female energy in the body to ease your physical and emotional pain. I will focus on both the right side of the body, female energy and on the left side of the body, male energy.

The small muscle that sits in between the clavicle bone and spine of scapula, in between the shoulder girdle, found on the top of both sides of your shoulder, is wrapped over by the trapizius muscle. Here you will find your immediate family members. From the end of the shoulder to two inches in on the right side, this is where sister/s, daughter/s, granddaughter/s can be found. Take your fingers and press into the soft part of this muscle, pain here indicates difficulties or worries in any of these relationships. Move your fingers further down the line where the neck meets the shoulder, this is known as the mother corner and would be your relationship with your mother in your adult life. Your grandmother/s is next to her. Press in this area and again, if tightness or knots are found it can reflect tricky, not easy, complicated issues with your mother or grandmother. If your relationship is good as an adult with either or both, then it can simply be you worrying about their health, coping with their loss or any other matter you have on your mind about them. If you move to the left side of the top of your shoulder and again, apply the same principles, you find on the end of the shoulder is where your brother/s, son/s, grandson/s would be, grandfather/s would follow and your father energy would be in the corner at the base of the neck. A knot of any kind here again would reflect difficulties in the relationship, worries or loss over father. **Diagram 4d** shows what I call 'the family collar', because the connection of muscles from shoulder to shoulder and its surrounding area is a compilation of our loved ones and are our most painful spots. The way in which it falls, resembles a collar on a blouse, it is our most concealed outfit, invisible to the human eye.

Diagram 4d

Family Collar

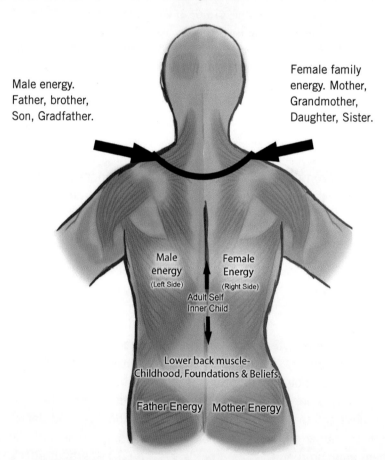

Male energy.
Father, brother,
Son, Gradfather.

Female family
energy. Mother,
Grandmother,
Daughter, Sister.

Male
energy
(Left Side)

Female
Energy
(Right Side)

Adult Self
Inner Child

Lower back muscle-
Childhood, Foundations & Beliefs.

Father Energy   Mother Energy

The neck represents two departments. If you are a female, the right side of your neck mirrors your stress, worries and how you are coping. Any worries or problems you have with your boyfriend, partner or husband will be shown on the left side of your neck. If you are a male, then the left side of the neck reflects your stress, worries and how you are coping at the time. The right side of your neck will reflect your relationship with your partner, girlfriend or wife. Any soreness, discomfort, knots in this area shows problems, difficulties, strains in the relationship or over concern for your partner over health or their job. It is a standing joke and widely used term that our partners can be 'a pain in the neck' whoever coined that phrase was ahead of their time. There are five pressure points in the muscle that you can massage lightly at the back of the head, just underneath the skull bone called the occipital. This will help to ease built up tension in this area and down the neck muscle. Works lovely when using blended lavender oil.

The 'Yang' Energy Collection

In Eastern medicine, yang, male energy, flows into none emotional elements of our lives. In other words, it governs various genre's such as our work, education, health, bereavement, divorce, changes in the home renovation or move, justice, court, council, government, finance, travel in the UK and overseas. It is found on the left side of the back, on the trapezius muscle, from the side of the scapula bone (shoulder blade) and runs 6 inches down the muscle. Pain from this area shows changes in all or some of these fields You will know instantly whether you have recently lost a loved one, be worrying over financial matters or health issues, suffered travel delays, problems with education or the law. Whatever, pain comes from this area means a negative connection, it is your worry building and producing knots. I call this large group of subjects the Yang collection because it is always found on the male side, which is Yang energy. For the majority of people I see and treat, they will always have a small group forming here because we are always going to have something going on in one of those areas in our life. **Diagram 5e** reflects all the above locations in our body. Please use this to help determine any blockages you may feel in your muscles and what they may link to. Look at what is currently going on in your life or has been worrying you over the past 12 months or more.

Diagram 5e

Back of Body

Parent

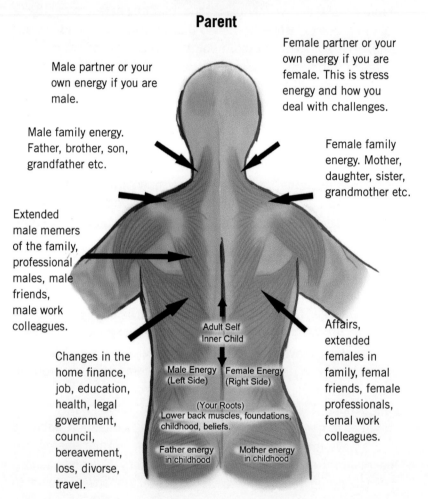

Male partner or your own energy if you are male.

Female partner or your own energy if you are female. This is stress energy and how you deal with challenges.

Male family energy. Father, brother, son, grandfather etc.

Female family energy. Mother, daughter, sister, grandmother etc.

Extended male memers of the family, professional males, male friends, male work colleagues.

Affairs, extended females in family, femal friends, female professionals, femal work colleagues.

Changes in the home finance, job, education, health, legal government, council, bereavement, loss, divorse, travel.

Adult Self
Inner Child

Male Energy (Left Side)

Female Energy (Right Side)

(Your Roots)
Lower back muscles, foundations, childhood, beliefs.

Father energy in childhood

Mother energy in childhood

THE WAY FORWARD

Being more aware of how our muscles store our emotional pain, helps you understand more about how our physical pain is created. Yes it takes more than just daily stress to produce acute and chronic back pain; there are other lifestyle factors to take into consideration. Look at the following list of questions and answer as honestly as you can;

- How much water do you drink daily?
- Do you have a more active or sedentary life?
- How much do you move each day using exercise, walking or rebounding?
- How much of your diet is processed?
- How much sugar do you take including those hidden in your diet?
- Are you overweight for your age and height?
- Are you moody, stressed or both?
- Do you like who you see in the mirror, dressed and undressed?

Depending on how you answered will determine your physical pain. Each of the above contributes to an imbalance in your body. I'm not getting you to become a perfect, model human being; I am getting you to understand that all of the above will add to your pain gauge. I go into more detail in the chapters that follow, but will briefly touch as to why now.

How much water do you drink – in my first book I wrote about the importance of keeping hydrated. When we don't drink enough water, primarily the best form of hydration, decaffeinated drinks such as herbal teas are good, but water rules supreme, we start to shrivel. Like a plant or tree needs water to thrive, so do we. Our brain suffers lapses of concentration when we do not take enough water on board; we feel tired and have a lack of energy in our body. Our spine is like our stem that supports our back. The spine also protects your spinal cord. The spinal cord is the column of nerves that connects your brain with the rest of your body, allowing you to control your movements. Without a spinal cord, you could not move any part of your body and your organs could not function. That is why keeping your spine healthy is vital if you want to live an active life. The spine is made up of 24 small bones each bone is called vertebrae. In between each vertebra is a soft gel-like cushion called a disc. The discs help absorb pressure and keep the bones from rubbing against each other. When the discs become dehydrated, like any sponge they become rigid and shrink, closing the gap between the vertebrae. Pressure starts to be felt in various parts of the back radiating out to the surrounding muscles. Equally, extremely tight locked back muscles, can work against the spine, like a pressure cooker and long term build up can force spinal problems to develop. As we age our discs lose water content, it becomes even more essential that we drink enough water daily to keep our discs hydrated to prevent further damage.

Do you have a more active or sedentary life – too many hours sat down will create its own problems. Whether its sat at your desk at home or work for long spells or on the couch, your body will get used to using the same muscles and through muscle memory, repetitive posture positions begin to form and we get more 'wear and tear' in those areas. Taking regular breaks hourly ensures your muscles break that pattern. I don't need an excuse for a lovely cup of Yorkshire tea or refreshing glass of water. Getting a breath of fresh air for 5 minutes outside has been proven to stimulate our senses and give us a natural energy boost.

How much do you move each day using exercise, walking or rebounding – I have dedicated chapter's 6 and 7 of this book to explain why this is very important so I won't spill the beans till you get there.

How much of your diet is processed? How much sugar do you take including those hidden in your diet? Are you overweight for your age and height? Are you moody, stressed or both? Do you

like who you see in the mirror, dressed and undressed – we can put all these points in one category as they all interlink with each other. If you eat a more processed, fatty and sugary diet, you will put on weight. When you carry more weight, this is added pressure on your skeletal system and referral pain starts to bleed into your joints and then echoes into the muscles. The heavier you become the more you don't like looking at yourself in the mirror. You start to feel moody as your clothes don't fit right. Certain areas become more expanded, like the waistline, love handles develop and muffin tops form, sounds like a cookery class. We become frustrated, angry to the point we begin to ignore the S.O.S signals our body sends out. Yes we work against ourselves, the more we know something is not good for us, the more we crave it and it becomes a never ending vicious circle. I know this circle well, as I have been part of the 'small big, big small' cycle for at least three decades of my life. For all the support and advice you are given by family members or experts, you prefer to turn your back on it (excuse the pun) and choose to blame the event, challenges and people in your life to justify your behaviour and reaffirm that it was these events, that caused you to become the way you are now, it's not your fault really is it? This way of thinking is your inner child coming to the rescue, recognise how your mini me jumps to your adult defence, remember you are a team after all. This is the same behaviour pattern a five year old would display in the playground in primary school. The 'she's not playing because...' 'He's not joining our gang' routine.

We are like yoyo's we go up and down with fluctuating diets, excuses, irregular exercise patterns ever seeking to hit our target which is more balance, happiness, peace, value, respect and love, but putting little effort in to achieving it means you will always fail, are we so not worth it? Getting to know you is your prime responsibility. When you get to know the you in you, you will feel free and easy, ready to change for the better. Over the coming chapters I will show you how to move forward, I give you simple proven processes that work and are easy to introduce into your lifestyle. Rome wasn't built in a day, but you have to start one day to make that change, why not sooner than later.

NATURAL PAIN SOLUTIONS

Upper and Middle Back Pain, controlled by your adult energy & Lower Back Pain controlled by your inner child –

Solution

When family issues or events from childhood manifest as neck, shoulder and back pain, dealing with them can be emotionally intense, the following exercises will give you instant stress release. Once you feel calmer, you can identify the emotions, memories or people in your life that are causing you stress and then take steps to deal with them.

Just breathe – Take a breath in to a count of four, then breathing out to a count of seven. Repeat this at least six times and notice how much better you feel. Breathing out for a longer period than you breathe in triggers the relaxation response.

Clear Your Head – Place the fingers of both hands on your forehead, halfway between the hairline and your eyes. Massage your skin upwards and backwards in small circles. Now place your thumbs on your temples, next to your eyes. Keep this position for at least five minutes, breathing deeply, until you feel calm.

Cut the Cords – Cords are the invisible energetic connection between people. At the end of each day, tune in to your body and try to sense if there is anyone who is tugging at you. Visualise where the cord is attached to you and imagine cutting it with a pair of scissors. Feel free.

Throat – controlled by your adult energy

This is your communication centre if physical symptoms occur they would be sore throat, tonsillitis, thyroid problems. Emotional reaction an inability to articulate your feelings, resentment, low self-esteem.

In Eastern philosophy, the throat is linked to communication, creativity and self expression. People with an underactive thyroid are often listless or quiet and don't speak much. They tend to harbour resentment and hold in what they really want to say. Those with overactive thyroid tend to be more outgoing and extroverted, but they also talk too much. In both cases, there is an imbalance.

Solution

As your confidence increases your throat energy should rebalance. Work out what it is that you're not expressing with this writing exercise. Make time to sit quietly for 15 minutes, then write these headings on a sheet of paper;

- **What is it I'm not saying?** - For example, are you frustrated that a partner, colleague or friend is taking you for granted?
- **Why am I allowing this?** – Are you afraid of a partner's anger or indifference? That your friend will be annoyed if you speak up? That you don't want to rock the boat at work?
- **What would I like to say or ask for?** – Think about the changes that would make you happier, such as being able to leave work on time or for your needs to be acknowledged.
- **What would happen if I voiced how I feel?** –What's the worst possible result? What's stopping you?
- **What actions can I take to break old patterns?** – Make one change in how you express yourself. For example, next time a friend expects you to do her a last minute favour, say no as politely and firmly as possible. This is you supporting your boundaries.

Heart & Chest- controlled by your adult energy

Solution
Practice daily meditation. You've tried and found it difficult? Here

are some easy mini meditations on how to succeed without over challenging yourself and healing your heart at the same time;

1. Try the 100 breaths technique.

Take 100 breaths. Count them. Try not to think about anything else.

This gives your brain something to do while the rest of you is relaxing through the meditating.

2. Take a meditation nap.

Lie down on a bed, couch, or sun lounge.

Close your eyes and do nothing. If your body naturally falls asleep allow it. You'll just happily float along. Put a lovely peace of relaxing music on and drift for 10 minutes. Meditation should be enjoyable.

3. Use the alarm clock meditation.

Set a timer for five minutes. Then meditate until the timer goes off. This way, you don't have to wonder about how long it's been, or how much longer you should meditate for. It's like meditation on cruise-drive.

4. Get comfortable.

When you start your meditation you should be as relaxed and comfortable as possible. If you are not, then your focus will be on how uncomfortable you are sitting. Meditating isn't an exercise in feeling uncomfortable. It's a place of rest, stillness and comfort. So get comfy.

5. Start small.

When you a pushed for time and really would like to meditate but feel under too much pressure, simply stop and take ten breaths. Then if it feels good take another ten or twenty breaths. If you feel refreshed enough stop there, if not take another ten or twenty till you do.

Start small. Everyone has time for 10 breaths. See what happens. It's a little way of moving around resistances.

6. Make it a reward.

Meditation should be fun and easy, and it should feel good for you, not excruciatingly boring or painful. Work out the thing about meditation that makes it really, really useful for you. Not "I should meditate because everyone says so." Not even an "I should meditate."Find a way that makes you think, "I want to meditate."

Whenever I take 100 breaths, it may be boring for the first half but after that, it feels like nirvana. I don't know if it's a rush of oxygen to the head or just because I finally relax then, but whatever it is, the second half is good. It makes the beginning so very, very worth it. My little reward is the second-half release. Find your personal treat from meditating. And keep remembering it. Use it as a reward for getting yourself there.

7. Use help when you need it.

If you need extra help in meditating, use CDs. They're like little personal guides into sweet-calm-space.

Try out different CDs, guides, and meditation techniques, and see what works for you. Don't think you have to go it alone. Everything's easier with a little support.

8. And most of all…

Remember that the reason you aren't meditating right now is not because you are lazy. It's because you haven't yet found a way to meditate for you that is fun, easy, and comfortable for you. Find the way that does, and then it's much, much easier.

Remove the annoying parts from meditating. Try out all the different ways you can to make it as lovely an experience as possible.

And remember: you are the expert on you. Find the wonderful things that work for you, and ignore the rest.

Legs, Knees & Feet- controlled by your inner child

Physical symptoms are Rheumatism, knee problems, poor circulation. Emotional symptoms worry, fears about basic survival, anxiety. In Eastern philosophy, the legs and feet are ruled by the root chakra, at the base of our spine. This is where our foundations are found, this is known as the survival centre and reveals how secure you feel.

Solution

Learn to ground yourself through a walking meditation as follows;

To balance the root chakra you need to stand barefoot on grass or earth not concrete which will connect you to the healing and grounding energy of the earth's vibration. As you do so, close your eyes and breathe deeply and slowly. Visualise the earth's energy entering through your feet and filling you with strength. Walk barefoot for 10-15 minutes. For the first 30 seconds focus on the sounds around you, like the birds singing or the rustling of leaves. For the next 30 seconds, focus on the smells around you, such as the scent of flowers, grass or smoke in the air. Finally, notice any physical sensations, such as the warmth of the sun on your bare skin or a cool breeze. It could even be the sensation of your soles touching the ground with each step. After a few minutes, notice how your body feels. Do you feel lighter and more relaxed? Practice this walking mediation regularly to help you feel calmer and more grounded and to experience the range of health benefits earth's energy can bring.

MEASURE YOUR WORTH

Another simple exercise in releasing back pain, created by emotional disconnection between the inner child and adult, is finding out where you are in the 'care giving' queue. How many times do you give in to doing things for others, when you really wanted the time for your needs. How many times did you cancel your plans to make someone else happy? Get two small or medium glass jars with screw on lids. Every time you cancel what you are doing to please or help someone else unplanned, pop a copper coin like a 2p piece in one of the jars. Every time you stick to your plans and do something nice for you, pop a silver or gold coin in the other jar, like 50p or £1 coin. Soon you will visually see which jar grows the quickest and will be able to determine where you are in the 'care giving' queue for you. If you fill the copper jar first, this will indicate that you put yourself last most of the time and naturally cancel things last minute to help others. That's all well and good, but will frustrate your inner child as you always keep him/her in the corner, they never go out to play. If you fill the gold or silver coin jar first, this represents you putting yourself first, you can either donate it to your favourite charity, or go and treat yourself to something nice, like a pamper treatment, skincare product or piece of dress jewellery. Then you can be reminded that you are worth it. If you don't want to use coins, you can fill one jar with your favourite sweets and the reward is eating them at the end. The other jar you fill with all the sweets you don't like, because if you fill this jar first, you can give it away to those you put first, like you give your time away so freely.

5

SUGAR

'The candy man can cos he mixes it with love and
makes the world taste good'

'The Candy Man' song by Sammy Davis Jr

In order to conquer back pain, any pain, we need to look at all the contributory factors in our lifestyle that can affect our physical and emotional wellbeing. How much balance we have in all three areas, in what we eat, drink and how we move, has a significant influence on our fitness. You cannot ignore the fact that each plays an important part in your mental and physical health. Too much sugar in your diet for instance, can make you moody, tired, irritable and not able to think clearly leading to a negative state untreated, this can eventually trigger depression. In this chapter I would like you to understand how sugar really changes your life for the worse and leave you one step closer to recognising that life would be much better without it.

In the earliest years of my childhood, I grew up in a time when chocolate, sweets, biscuits and cakes were seen as a luxury. They made their appearance on birthdays, Easter, Christmas and special occasions, which were when my parents entertained friends for dinner. Out would come the dessert tray filled with a Victoria sandwich sponge, selection of half coated chocolate covered biscuits and a box of after dinner mints which I thought yuck at the time, but desperate times made a 7 year old me appreciate their value. Even growing up in a time when sugar was scarce in our household, in my early years of the 1960's we were slim, healthy children living on good old classic homemade dishes with plenty of fresh fruit, veg and water. Then came the 1970's and my father moved out of his factory job, qualified after studying years at night school as a T.V engineer and suddenly, we escalated from a poor to middle class family to middle to high class status. His job came with a company car and extra money, which contributed to more luxurious items including extra shopping. My parents came to England in the late 1950's both had experienced loss and starvation from the Second World War. My mum was an excellent cook and extremely thrifty, she could turn a piece of pig skin into a first class dish fit for any restaurant critic, so the extra income was more than welcome. My father had a very generous side to him which led at times to him squandering his hard earned cash on unnecessary white goods, such as a state of the art Hammond organ, nobody could play, but he liked it, so became self taught to justify the £3,000 price tag. He loved the expansion of the new local supermarket on our doorstep Morrisons, he would always be popping in to top up the shop with treats for us as well as himself. Biscuits, cakes and sweets become the norm from the age of 9 upwards in our household. Suddenly, we had a pop man turn up every week on our doorstep. Dad would shout 'the Alpine pop man is here, what flavours do you want.' All three children charged to the wagon to look at the lovely coloured pop bottles with the most bizarre flavours. Each week we all got to choose one flavour, but we could drink what we wanted, plus there was dad's choice and even though my mother never drank any pop in her lifetime, dad would drink her share and choose two flavours himself. So we all carried into the kitchen five one litre bottles of fizzy pop a week. Most new flavours had and 'ade' added to it like, Limeade, Raspberryade, Strawberryade, Pineappleade, then there was also the classic Dandelion & Burrdock, Cream Soda, Cola and Lemonade the list was endless.

My point being in all of this is that sugar surrounds all of us, it devours our life, infiltrates every food we eat and drink we drink. It is hard to get away from, is it any wonder we are all slaves to its taste. It's our silent killer, it's one of the main reasons we have become such an obese nation, its ageing our skin, our body and creating disease, yet we entertain it every day in our diet. I search my own history for when this innocent addiction began and it did begin innocently. Our parents and generations before them were all naive in understanding the hidden dangers behind sugar. Their ignorance of knowledge was not their fault, if they knew then what we know now, they would have had a very different approach in how they introduced it into our lives, or would they? Dipping baby's dummies into sugar was a common way to keep a baby happy and quiet. Yes it would keep baby quiet, as the child sucked on the sucrose, its taste buds learning a new sensation that entered its blood stream. That amount of sugar, no matter how small in relation to the baby, enters its blood stream and releases insulin. As baby is not using any of this sugar stored energy, as it is only weeks or months old, it's only at the wriggling gurgling stage; baby falls asleep within five minutes. To me it's like giving your child a line of cocaine, you would never dream of doing it. I know as soon as I have eaten a bar of chocolate, I will be a sleep on my couch within ten minutes as my body is not used to so much sugar in one hit. The more your body gets used to it, the higher the quantity it needs to knock you out. A bit like an alcoholic, the more they drink the more the body adapts to it, so it can cope with a higher dose.

With all the information saturating the market about how sugar harms us, what it does to us, all the arguments for and against we still can't stop ourselves loving it, craving it, needing it, wanting it and demanding it. There are good things it gives us such as energy, but they are minor in comparison to the harm it does to our cells. What has sugar to do with back pain I hear you murmur. Well sorry to disappoint you, but it can only be bad news. I have the 'person who snatched the dummy from the baby's mouth' feeling coming over me, like I'm the bad guy delivering the following information, but here goes anyway, you need to know the truth about sugar. For those who already know this stuff forgive me, but the repetition is worth it I promise.

SUGAR INDUCED INFLAMMATION

Sugar can also cause back pain - Fact. If you drink too many soft drinks in a day, the excess sugar can cause severe pain in the back. Oh, you don't drink soft drinks, that's good, but the equivalent found in your daily foods which are hidden sugars equate to the same. Our diets are sugar loaded, sneaked in to most recipes to tickle our taste buds as we learnt from being babies. Popular foods are;

- Sweets, chocolate, fizzy drinks, baked pies & cakes, pizza, ice cream, crackers, ketchup, biscuits, bread, yogurts are loaded with sugar and often, high fructose corn syrup. Then there are pasta, potatoes and white rice and alcohol which turn into sugar in our body.
- Of the 100 to 180 pounds of sugar we consume each year, less than 30 pounds are from the sugar bowl. The rest comes from foods and soft drinks.

As little as 2 teaspoons of sugar can off set your body chemistry and unbalance homeostasis. Our bodies have a unique balance needed to be able to repair and maintain life. Inflammation is one of the ways our immune system responds to assault or injury. When we consume too much sugar, our body releases insulin and stress hormones. These in turn trigger the inflammation process. The places where we have the least circulation of the blood, we have the greatest risk of inflammation. This is why our joints and especially our back is at greatest risk.

OUR HUMAN FISH POND

The average human body is composed of approximately 72 trillion cells. Each cell is programmed to perform a specific function. The ability to perform a required task is solely dependent on the health of that cell.

A human cell is much like a small pond and its fragile ecosystem. The cell is a small pool of water surrounded on all sides by a border. The border surrounding the human tissue cell is a protective coating of fats and proteins. The protective coating allows various substances into the cellular pond. Suspended in the cell's fluid (the cellular pond) are numerous small organs called organelles. The organelles rely on the nutrients that cross the protective cell wall to supply the raw materials and energy needed to perform that cell's specific task. The process occurs in much the same way that the fish in the small pond rely on the stream's flow into the pond.

A POLLUTED POND

If the stream that flows into a pond becomes polluted with toxic substances, the pond will not be able to support life for very long. The human cell is much the same. When toxic (such as sugar) or abnormal substances are allowed across the cell wall, the normal functioning of the cell is distracted and slowed. As the cell becomes more and more polluted, its function slows and the cell dies. When a great enough number of the cells that constitute an organ die, then the organ becomes painful and eventually diseased. When a body part, such as the muscle in the back becomes painful, the part struggles to heal and repair itself. Much of the pain experienced during a chronic neck, shoulder and lower back pain cycle is generated by tissue damage, inflammation and cellular pollution.

When I was out in Hawaii in 2000 with the Anthony Robbins Academy training to be an NLP Practitioner, I learnt how damaging sugar can be to our cells. We all had our fingers pricked and placed a blob of blood on a slide to view our cells on day one under a microscope. I could see that certain cells, in fact most of my cells were moving really slowly and actually sticking together in two's or three's. This was a reflection of how much sugar was in my blood stream and its affect on the performance of my cells. This was not a good sign, as ideally they should be swimming around like sperm, fast doing their job efficiently carrying nutrients to all parts of my body, including my vital organs. I was rather disappointed to see even a slim person like myself was not as great on the inside as I had originally thought. Throughout the 14 day course of continual study, we were encouraged to drink alkalised water which would improve the ph level in the body, making you feel more energised, able to concentrate better and be pain free. After just 24 hours of drinking alkalised water we were asked to re-do the blood test. I was amazed to see my cells running around like little ants busying themselves, what a difference a day made. I continued to drink alkalised water for a good six months on my return, but like every great habit, Christmas came and it got broke.

WHERE YOU STAND WITH THE WHITE STUFF

White table sugar (sucrose) greatly increases pain - this is especially true for sufferers of back pain, spinal arthritis and fibromyalgia. You might not take it direct in tea's coffees but it is present in most of your food and drink in hidden forms disguised under different names. Sugar's impact on pain is probably linked to the mineral loss associated with diets high in refined sugar. Human muscle relies on the minerals calcium, magnesium, potassium and sodium for smooth and coordinated contraction and relaxation. A diet high in sugar causes the kidneys to extract calcium, magnesium and potassium from the blood and dump the minerals into the urine. The body then scavenges its bones and muscles to make up the mineral deficiency in the blood. The process results in muscles already less flexible due to back pain becoming even more aggravated. Since sugar causes the body to extract minerals from bone and muscle, it's logical that sugar consumption intensifies pain.

Eating sugar also creates another problem for those suffering from back pain and arthritis, sugar directly increases inflammation. When sugar is eaten, the human body will either use it for blood sugar or convert it into fat for storage. Sugar is readily converted into a bad fat, namely saturated fat. Saturated fat is a problem for back pain sufferers because it contains the fatty acid arachidonic acid. Arachidonic acid is converted by arthritic joint tissues into an inflammatory substance called a series two prostaglandin. The conversion of sugar to saturated fat increases the amount of arachidonic acid available and results in an increase in inflammation and pain. Saturated fat also builds around the waistline, adds to belly fat. The bigger your belly, the more you lose your core strength. Losing core strength will add to your back pain, in particularly your mid to lower back.

One solution is to eat less sugar or cut it out altogether. Since lifestyle sometimes does not allow us to control our diet as we would like, water provides a good option in offering a temporary cure. It will help dilute insulin which will reduce any inflammation. The best water is alkalised water, which is easy to make as there are now hundreds of green alkalising powders on the market today. Just add a teaspoon in a litre of filtered water shake and you are good to go. Small change big difference, within days you'll go through a small detox as the alkalisation process cleans all your body out of toxic build up, but the result is simply great. More energy, clearer head, no pain! How good is that, a natural way to get rid of pain without the need for prescription drugs. Too good to be true? Try it and see for yourself. As with any new change you have to ensure its ok with your GP first, especially if you are on strong medication or high painkillers it does change the status quo in your body, like fine tuning a car. You may not be able to go through a mini detox, so please check next time you are at the doctors.

SUGAR CONDITIONING

From babies we are learning the taste sensation of sugar from our dummies coated in the nasty white stuff. This explosion continues throughout our childhood, puberty, young adulthood and so on. Let's play a memory game. I'll ask you to think of any year, month or day in your life and I can guarantee, that's if you don't cheat which I'm sure you won't, that you will be able to recall your favourite sugar related memoir. For instance, as a child we spent many a summer taking day trips to the East coast, visiting the seaside town of Scarborough, a family favourite. I could guarantee an ice cream on the beach, a donkey ride and a visit to one of the hundreds of rock shops on the promenade. I loved the rock shops, it was filled with every colour rock, a minty hard confectionary made of 100% pure sugar and water crystallised to form hard rock. The rock would be moulded into all shapes and sizes. My favourite was the sugar dummy, a perfect replica of a baby's dummy, but four times the size with a lovely ribbon to hang round your neck, now where did they get that idea from? Camping visits to the Lake District would always mean a large block of Kendal mint cake to share, another specialised confectionary similar to rock, but softer. Back home, regular bank holidays saw the fun fair come to town and cinder toffee with candy floss was our treat. Bonfire night we all enjoyed toffee apples, cinema trips equalled popcorn, playing out every night during the summer holidays called for a 99 ice cream from the ice cream man. Christmas time was filled with sweet stockings and selection boxes. Easter brought no Easter bunny, but Easter eggs for sure, most children averaged about 15 medium size eggs enough chocolate to last six months, but usually gone within the week and not a chocolate crispy insight. How well did you do with your sugar memory, I'm sure the list is endless.

Advertising, film and music over the decades have also been a massive driving force behind our sugar fest. In the 1970's Ribena was seen as the best drink to give your children for strong healthy teeth and bones fortified with all the necessary minerals they needed and no family, including ours, was seen without it, 100% pure sugar even though it was diluted. Breakfast cereals all came with a free toy and many were miniature collectables. This was the way manufacturers aimed at encouraging children to eat breakfast and increase their sales. Adding essential nutrients and minerals to the products helped convince parents they making the right choice for their family, ignoring the ingredients list through ignorance and how many spoons of sugar each serving gave.

My favourite film was the 1971 hit 'Willy Wonka and the Chocolate Factory.' I wanted to enter that factory and scoff all those delicious treats and swim in the milk chocolate river. It was such a success they remade it again in 2005, with Johnny Depp playing Mr Wonka and they even brought out a West End Musical in 2013 for another generation to enjoy, including my children, educating future generations into loving the sweetie world. Childhood memories of sugar connects with our inner child. Chocolates, ice cream was seen as a treat or reward. If you wanted to fit in with your peers, you all had to have a sweet treat at playtime. As most children in the late 60's and early 70's walked to school, they would buy something on the way to school and flash their goodies off at playtime. If you didn't have anything to show, you didn't play with them, it was as simple as that, sugar opened doors for you. On the way home, you always had time for day dreaming and a gobstopper gave you endless sucking time, to sweeten the dream.

When you try and break your addiction from sugar, during a detox diet for instance, you are killing the habit to the inner childs memory as well. So breaking it can be a two way battle. Another family film was the 1968 British Musical 'Chitty Chitty Bang Bang' a scene with the child catcher tempting the children out of the house with his sweets and lollipops. In the musical 'Oliver' again we hear the boys singing about 'Food glorious food' and see them grabbing sweets, chocolate, desserts as if that is all part of the healthy process of the food chain. What about the lovely Julie Andrews as 'Mary Poppins', convincing us that a spoon full of sugar helps the medicine go down and it did. It also triggers a multitude of problems later in life and tooth decay. I know I'm knit picking now, but I want to highlight how these sublime messages surround us daily and ingrain in our brain, reassuring us that sugar is safe, it's ok. Yes it is if controlled, but we don't control it do we?

Every morning I listen to one of my favourite shows on Radio 2 with the great Chris Evans. Chris puts together with his team, a wonderful fun filled and very entertaining programme, that puts a spring in your step for the rest of the day. One of his regular tunes played during the week is Sammy Davis Jr's 'The Candy Man' song, a firm favourite of mine. Another great song that tells us that 'the Candy Man can cause he mixes it with love and makes the world taste good.' Enforcing that sugar (candy man) makes the world taste good, so without it life is bad. We are bathed daily in such messages from advertising bill boards, adverts in magazines, newspapers, posters. Radio and T.V advertising, supermarket promotions. Why is it that all the 3 for 2 offers are mainly on sugar loaded drinks or food? The more sugar we eat daily the more the addiction takes hold, the more it creates our world of pain, obesity, belly fat, heart disease and much more. We are selling to our children and the next generation, the message that sugar is king, sugar is safe and energising. We have a back catalogue of celluloid films and music to support that message. What we really should be saying is, yes it is safe in moderation, but if you take more than a spoon a day, be prepared to accept what comes with it.

THE TRUTH ABOUT SUGAR

Our relationship with sugar is like a lifelong marriage with zero effort made, it has its ups and downs, but eventually will cost you. Excessive sugar in the diet is not the best idea when it comes to healthy living. Nonetheless, few of us are consuming sugar in sensible amounts; most of us are eating tons of it. In fact, worldwide we are consuming about 500 extra calories per day from sugar. That's just about what you would need to consume if you wanted to gain a pound a week. Most people know that sugar is not good for them, but for some reason, they think the risk of excess sugar consumption is less than that of having too much saturated and trans fat, sodium or calories. Perhaps it's sugar's lack of sodium or fat that make it the "lesser of several evils," or perhaps people are simply of the mind frame that what they don't know won't hurt them. If you really knew what it was doing to your body, though, you might just put it at the top of your "foods to avoid" list. Here are a few things that may surprise you about sugar.

Sugar can damage your heart

While it's been widely noted that excess sugar can increase the overall risk for heart disease, a 2013 study from the Journal of the American Heart Association displayed strong evidence that sugar can actually affect the pumping mechanism of your heart and could increase the risk for heart failure. The findings specifically pinpointed a molecule from sugar (as well as from starch) called glucose metabolite glucose 6-phosphate (G6P) that was responsible for the changes in the muscle protein of the heart. These changes could eventually lead to heart failure. Approximately half of the people that are diagnosed with heart failure die within five years. My father was one such victim, so I understand this disease well. No heart disease in our family, but due to his ignorance of the facts about sugar he saw it as a harmless, pleasant substance that eventually cost him his life.

Sugar specifically promotes belly fat

Obesity in general has tripled in the past 30 years and childhood obesity rates have doubled. Many of us are aware of the data that demonstrates just how literally big our future is looking, but beyond the studies and all the initiatives to curb childhood obesity, one needs only to visit an amusement park, school or shopping centres to truly see what is happening. One factor that seems to inflict obese children is fat accumulation in the trunk area of the body. Why? One cause may be the increase in sugar-laden beverages. A 2010 study in children found that excess sugar intake (but not glucose intake) actually caused visceral fat cells to mature setting the stage for a big belly and even bigger future risk for heart disease and diabetes.

Sugar is the true silent killer

Move over salt and hypertension, you've got competition. Sugar, as it turns out, is just as much of a silent killer. A 2008 study found that excess sugar consumption was linked to an increase in a condition called leptin resistance. Leptin is a hormone that tells you when you've had enough food. The problem is, we often ignore the signal our brain sends to us. For some people though, leptin simply does not want to work, leaving the person with no signal whatsoever that the body has enough food to function. This in turn can lead to over consumption of food and consequently, obesity. Why the silent killer? Because it all happens without symptoms or warning bells. If you've gained weight in the past year and can't quite figure out why, perhaps you should look at how much sugar you're feeding your body.

Your sugar "addiction" may be genetic

If you've ever said, "I'm completely addicted to sugar," you may actually be correct. A recent study of 579 individuals showed that those who had genetic changes in a hormone called ghrelin consumed more sugar (and alcohol) than those that had no gene variation. Ghrelin is a hormone that tells the brain you're hungry. Researchers think that the genetic components that effect your ghrelin release may have a lot to do with whether or not you seek to enhance a neurological reward system through your sweet tooth.

Sugar and alcohol have similar toxic liver effects on the body

A 2012 paper in the journal *Nature*, suggested that limitations and warnings should be placed on sugar similar to warnings we see on alcohol and cigarette packets. The authors showed evidence that sugar and glucose in excess can have a toxic effect on the liver as the metabolism of ethanol the alcohol contained in alcoholic beverages had similarities to the metabolic pathways that sugar took. Further, sugar increased the risk for several of the same chronic conditions that alcohol was responsible for. Finally, if you think that your slim stature keeps you immune from sugar causing liver damage, think again. A 2013 study found that liver damage could occur even without excess calories or weight gain.

Sugar is ageing you & may sap your brain power

When I think back on my childhood; I remember consuming more sugar than I probably should have. I should have enjoyed my youth back then, because unfortunately, all the sugar may have accelerated the ageing process. A 2009 study found a negative relationship between sugar consumption and the ageing of our cells. Ageing of the cells consequently can be the cause of something as simple as wrinkles to something as dire as chronic disease. The more sugar you consume the faster your cells age. But there is other alarming evidence that sugar may affect the ageing of your brain as well. A 2012 study found that excess sugar consumption was linked to deficiencies in memory and overall cognitive health. A 2009 study in rats showed similar findings. With Dementia and Alzheimer's on the increase, could this be another link to the reason why.

Sugar hides in many everyday "non-sugar" foods

While many of us strive to avoid the "normal" sugary culprits (sweets, cookies, cake, etc.), they often are fooled when they discover some of their favourite foods also contain lots of sugar. Examples include tomato sauce, fat free dressing, tonic water, marinades, crackers and even bread. You have to be more vigilant when you shop, which in turn becomes more time consuming and time is what we all don't have these days. Maybe online shopping for food has its benefits, as you have more time in the comfort of your own home to browse through the ingredients list and make improved choices.

Sugar is making us fat

I figured I'd leave the most obvious fact for last. While you may be aware that too many calories from any source will be stored as fat if not burned, what you may not connect is that the lack of other nutrients in sugar actually makes it much easier to eat mouth full's of, with no physical effects to warn us of the danger that lurks. Foods rich in fibre, fat and protein all have been associated with increased fullness. Sugar will give you the calories, empty calories, but not the feeling that you've had enough. That's why you can have an entire king-size bag of extra sweet sugar coated popcorn (with its sky high glycemic index) at the movies and come out afterwards ready to go for dinner.

On a final note, it's important to point out that simple sugars from milk (in the form of lactose) don't display the same negative health effects that we see in studies when reviewing sugar's effects on the body. Simple sugars coming from fruit are also less concerning given their high amounts of disease-fighting compounds and fibre.

So now you know, and knowing perhaps can create action. You can do something about decreasing your overall sugar consumption without feeling deprivation or sheer frustration and in doing so win your war with back pain, all pain.

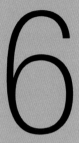

6

WALKING BACK TO HAPPINESS

'I'm bringing you love so true cause that's what I owe to you'

Sung by Helen Shapiro

I first heard this song played on my father's record player in 1969. It was a number one hit on its release in 1961. I was six years old and loved to dance to happy tunes and this was no exception, so it stayed in my good memories file. For those people who dislike exercise in the form of the 'gym' walking is a fabulous free alternative. What's all the fuss about walking I hear you say. Well every medic in the land encourages us to do it before any form of exercise and it's the first thing we learned to do after we crawled. We loved it as children, taking those first steps, what an adventure to escape our parents and make them run after us fretting to catch our falls. So why don't we love doing it so much now. For many of us do do it, but not enough are doing it. 21st century lifestyle allows us the luxury of great technology to create our sedentary lives. Cars, motorbikes, scooters, computers, laptops ipads, mobile phones, television, this explosion of techno gadgets have aided us in becoming a more obese nation, as well as token couch potatoes'. Again, I am not blaming technology I applaud it, but I am blaming the way we abuse it. Falling out of love with ourselves when we suddenly pile on the pounds is a result of a lack of movement. Too many calories and not enough activity equals being overweight it's not rocket science and every human understands this simple equation, so why keep on doing it. Emotional eating is the number one reason we binge on comfort foods, all processed with high calories, especially when feeling stressed. It's the love and connection we get from such foods that console our wounds and reassure our vulnerable state.

I've had many a pleasure visiting this state over the years, knowing at the time I was participating in the event of how wrong it was, but enjoying the moment of how right it felt at the time. Like a drug addict feeding their addiction. I needed my daily fix of cheese to meet what was lacking in my life, a loving relationship. I knew I had to break this pattern and my passion with cheese that gave me the unconditional love I was seeking. It's like taking a dummy away from a child; it's heartbreaking at the time because you know they can't sleep without it. It's their soother, but its doing their teeth no good and they need to stop relying on it for their own good. I successfully broke my habit with one 45 minute session of hypnotherapy. Hypnotherapy reprogrammed my mind messages and helped me stop the negative chatter of meeting my needs with cheese. In my peak I was eating my way through a block of mild cheddar cheese per night, what was I doing to my body I dare now not think! Like every story, mine does have a happy ending as I beat my demon. I now only eat cheese as a treat and not as a necessity.

What drives us towards this unhealthy lifestyle is the negative chatter of feeling undervalued, disrespected and unloved. The negative chatter is what we tell ourselves when our needs are not being met and the binging is triggered. This eventually leads to an increase in weight thus putting extra pressure on our muscles and skeletal system. Our body has to accommodate the extra person we are carrying around and over time it starts to release a signal called pain which is our body's cry for help. When we feel this pain we start to associate it with a physical action and frantically try to reason with ourselves whether we over did the driving, too long sat at the computer, got out of bed funny, but it's the excess weight, lack of mobility, that builds pressure in the our muscles with a sprinkling of negative emotional mindset that activates our muscle memory to retain pain. A large belly is another cause of back pain and loss of core strength. A bigger belly causes the pelvis to tilt out of alignment, with our body trying to maintain alignment; the back is put under a lot of strain. Pain can be felt in the lower back and travel down the legs referring in the knees. Walking will ease the pressure and help lose belly fat.

When I work at my London clinic in Harley Street I am forever mesmerised by the way people move. People watching is one of my favourite pastimes, though I make little time for it, when I do take five minutes and watch how people act in stores, on the streets towards our fellow man, it upsets me and at times, takes me by surprise. Simple tasks like crossing the road are made into life threatening risks. We are taught as children the rules of pedestrian crossing, to cross on the green man and wait at the side of the road when the red man shows. All the rules are broken when we become adults, if not earlier. I see people challenging the traffic, rushing to beat the mechanical machine, stepping in front of cars crossing on the red man, they don't make time to wait for the green man. I deliberately make myself wait even when there's no traffic, why, to give myself those few extra minutes of time, time to appreciate what I am doing, my surroundings, the weather. You may laugh thinking how strange, but it isn't, I am valuing my time for me, with me, do you do the same. Little pockets of time are lost every second of the day when we rush our dinner down, rush around the house getting dressed, life is just one big rush! Scheduling time for many people is a difficult thing to master, as they squeeze in everything they need to cram in and most of the time, it doesn't include what you like to do. So walking is a great way to make time for you. For those who dislike gyms, classes and more adventurous activities like cycling, triathlons or running, walking is time to get to know you, listen to the peace around you. It's a time that no one else can interrupt or intervene, as long as you put your mobile phone on silent. By being more active, moving more and reducing your portion intake by 25% you can achieve great weight loss and with weight loss comes less pain. The official footsteps count for a healthy lifestyle is 10,000 steps per day which adds up to 5 miles walking a day. So strap on a pedometer at the cost of a few pounds and from the minute you rise, to going to bed you will be able to see how many steps you actually take. The Step Diet, by James O. Hill, John C. Peters, Bonnie T. Jortberg, and Pamela Peeke, is a life-long program for both weight loss and weight maintenance. The easy-to-do plan helps dieters slowly increase their daily activity with the use of a pedometer that comes with the book. Even if you are slim, do not be fooled into thinking you don't have to exercise or move more, we all need to. Here are some of the most common questions my clients ask me about walking and its benefits.

WHAT'S SO GREAT ABOUT WALKING?

Walking can be done almost anywhere, at any time, and in any weather. It's a great way to get from A to B, which means you can fit walking into your daily routine. Walking is classed as a moderate-intensity activity and counts towards your recommended 150 minutes per week of exercise. If you walk 10,000 steps a day, you will probably do more than 150 minutes and that's great: research suggests that the more activity you do the better, as there are numerous benefits one being less pain.

HOW DO I KNOW HOW MANY STEPS I'M TAKING?

The average person walks between 3,000 and 4,000 steps per day. To find out how many steps you take each day, buy a pedometer. Clip it firmly to your belt or waist band and it will measure every step you take: around the house, across the office, window shopping, to school or the park. You might find that you walk almost 10,000 steps (about five miles a day) already, or that you walk less than you think. Whatever your results, knowing how far you can walk in a day will motivate you.

HOW MANY CALORIES WILL I BURN IF I WALK 10,000 STEPS A DAY?

A person aged 45 and weighing 70kg (about 11 stone) can burn around 400 calories by walking 10,000 steps briskly (3-5mph). If you're trying to lose weight, you should aim to burn 600 more calories than you take in through food and drink every day. This is best achieved by a combination of diet and exercise.

WHAT IF I DON'T DO ANY EXERCISE AT THE MOMENT?

If you're not very active, increase you're walking distances gradually. No one expects 10,000 steps on the first day! If you're worried about your joints or any existing health conditions, talk to your GP. If your joints are a problem, you can see if your local swimming pool holds exercise classes. The water helps to support your joints while you move, and once you lose a bit of weight, that will reduce the pressure on your joints. A few extra pounds around our middle, whether from indulgence or hormone imbalance, weight can cause pain so it's important to start walking the weigh off.

DO I NEED ANY SPECIAL CLOTHING?

A pair of cushioned trainers is recommended, which most people have already.

WHAT'S THE BEST WAY TO START?

Using your pedometer, find out how many steps you take during a normal day. It could be as little as 900 steps, or as many as 5,000 steps, depending on what you do. Record your daily steps over a week and use the total weekly number to work out a daily average. Use this daily average to build your steps gradually, by adding a few more steps every so often, until you're regularly walking 10,000 steps a day.

10,000 STEPS SOUNDS A LOT. HOW DO I FIT ALL THAT WALKING INTO MY BUSY DAY?

Increasing your walking is easier than you think. If you start with a negative approach you will avoid increasing your steps. Try these tips for getting more steps into your life:

- get off the bus early and walk the rest of the way home or to work
- walk to the station instead of taking the car or bus
- take the stairs instead of the lift, or walk up escalators
- invest in a shopping trolley and shop locally if you can
- walk the children to school, whatever the weather
- get fit by walking the dog

I FIND WALKING BORING. HOW CAN I MAKE IT MORE FUN?

- find a walking partner, so you have someone to chat to as you walk
- get an MP3 player and listen to your favourite music or podcasts as you go
- plan interesting walks during your days off
- join a walking group

HOW LONG DO I HAVE TO KEEP WALKING?

The rest of your life! Being active is a lifelong health habit. It's great for preventing weight gain, lifting your mood, decreasing pain and reducing your risk of many serious diseases, such as heart disease. It takes a while for a regular activity to become a healthy habit, so just keep going and it will become second nature. You'll soon find yourself doing many more than 10,000 steps on some days.

WHAT IF I CAN'T WALK FOR A FEW DAYS DUE TO ILLNESS OR A HOLIDAY?

Walking is a gentle form of exercise that is easy to get back into after a break. Just start again when you can, and build up slowly if you've been ill. The sooner you get back into the exercise groove, the better. When going on a holiday, choose one where you'll have plenty of opportunities to walk – for instance, along the beach or through the countryside.

IS WALKING ENOUGH? OR SHOULD I THINK ABOUT OTHER EXERCISE AS WELL?

If you're achieving at least 150 minutes of physical activity from walking, then you are meeting official health advice. If you want to add some variety to your activity, you could visit your local fitness centre and see what's on offer. Some people enjoy competitive sports, while others prefer sociable physical activity, such as dancing.

NEIL'S STORY

Neil was not only my client, but a very good friend for many years. I got to know him through a friend who recommended his services as a website designer. He was much more than that; Neil had many strings to his bow including being a fabulous cook, accomplished writer and painter. He was now in his mid 70's having gone through two heart bypasses and other health issues, was extremely overweight, suffering from a painful back as well as heavy legs. One day he couldn't stand the pain any longer, as it was restricting his mobility. He rarely ventured out of the house, did all his shopping online for home delivery and spent much of his day, sat down writing or painting. He needed to see the doctor desperately to get whatever medication he could prescribe to ease the pain in his muscles. The doctor listened attentively to Neil's list of physical symptoms ending with his plea for whatever tablet could take the problem away. The doctor spent a few minutes on his computer looking at the latest medication available, he scribbled on his pad and handed Neil the prescription. Neil glanced down to see if he recognised the drug, but was surprised to discover that the doctor did not give him one, two or any tablets. Instead what was written on the sheet was 'walk one mile a day.' Neil looked puzzled and pleaded with the doctor for something more tangible as it was a miracle he made it to the surgery that day. The doctor shook his head and reassured Neil that walking just one mile a day would not only ease his symptoms, but improve his total wellbeing. Neil left the surgery in disbelieve, but did as the doctor had told him. The next day he got in his car drove to the local park. He struggled to manage half a mile which took him best part of an hour and was wheezing throughout the exertion. The next day he went again, same time same place. After the first week he managed his first mile, he felt less breathless and took less than an hour. Three months later Neil lost 2 stone, still walks a mile a day, but now enjoys his morning walks, acknowledges other walkers and takes pictures of the park to paint. His pains had gone; he was a much healthier, happier, fitter man and all because he listened to his doctor and walked a mile a day.

THE IMPORTANCE OF BALANCING ENERGY

No matter how poor your mobility is, try and organise someone to walk with who can support you, if you are frail. Start with as little as 50 yards and build your target up to a mile a day. More steps saves lives, walking was a huge turning point in Neil's life. The need to bring more balance in all areas of diet and movement, will lead to an increase in improved health very rapidly, reducing or even eliminating your pain. It is our mind and the constant chatter that drives us to do the things we do.

The balancing of energy in our body is one part we must learn to master.

Why do we need to understand the importance of balancing male and female energy, Yin and Yang? Why do we need to be aware of this? This is not a new concept, it has an origin in eastern philosophies like Buddhism, Yoga and you can even find ancient writings that the Mayan civilization was aware of the power of maintaining balance between these two opposite energies.

Each human being has a right and left hemisphere in the brain, which we classify as male and female. The significant importance is that as one person we need to be in constant balance to be able to achieve the best of our world, mental, physical and emotional. Both sides, male and female have to attain a harmonious whole. When we experience blockages or imbalances within our male/female energy, the results can be disastrous and harmful to our physical body as well as our mental health. Introduce more walking into your world and you'll be surprised by the results you get and more.

7

BOUNCY! BOUNCY!

'Rubber ball I'll come bouncin' back to you'
Sung by Bobby Vee

REBOUNDING

In my first book I touched on the benefits of rebounding. I told you how I first discovered this wonderful form of exercise in 1983 whilst on a prospecting trip to Canada. I had seen my godfather bouncing on what looked like a child's mini trampoline. He told me it was a rebounder and he was using it as recommended by his heart surgeon, as part of his recovery programme from a heart bypass.

Yet again, I find myself writing about rebounding in my new book, because I cannot emphasis enough the positive almost 'life changing' affect it has on people's minds and bodies. I first used rebounding as part of my son's daily physiotherapy. Alex was born with Dextra Cardia Situs Inversus (all his internal organs reversed to ours) and 50% of those born with this rare condition have Primary Ciliary Dyskinesia (PCD), where the cilia hairs that line the nose, ears, and lungs don't work. Daily physiotherapy is essential to prevent regular respiratory infections; Alex found rebounding a fun way to conquer his regular physio routine. Now I was faced by another challenge, my mother.

MARIA'S STORY

My mother was approaching the tender age of 80 and since her unexpected heart bypass operation five years earlier, whilst also coming off HRT, old age suddenly took over her like a tsunami wave. Within weeks she had become 20 years older than her years. Then came the further diagnosis of COPD (Chronic Obstructive Pulmonary Disease attained from severe bouts of bronchitis and pneumonia over the years contracted from her job as a nurse, having never smoked). She physically looked herself, but it was her mobility that became extremely poor. This in turn led her to becoming more and more housebound. The less you go out, the more you become a prisoner of your environment. I recognised this battle as I had once been there, when I suffered from bouts of anxiety in my early 30's. It was extremely difficult to see my amazing mother, a wonder woman who had been a pillar of strength in my most difficult times, suddenly become so childlike and dependent on me. I think this is one of the hardest things we all have to face, not just our own old age, but for those still fortunate to have parents, seeing our parents go through this as well. Our inner child never wants to lose a parent or see a parent struggle; we want to remember them at their best. My mother never invested time in doing regular gym exercise and maintaining a positive outlook. She was always active and walked everywhere, which kept her physically slim, but that does not exempt you from all illnesses. She spent the majority of her life helping others, because of the conditioning she learnt as a child, she was a caring and dedicated nurse in the late 1970's and 80's, but also as a loving and self sacrificing parent. Her commitment to her work scarred her from her late forties, with lower back pain, due to lifting heavy patients. In Eastern medicine the lower back is your foundations and your childhood.

My Mother was an orphaned child from the age of 3, so lost her roots and childhood; her foundations were weak from the start. Raised in a convent by strict catholic nuns, she searched for love and connection by putting others before herself, only to always be met with disappointment and rejection. This in turn brought about a negative mindset pattern, which happens when humans encounter continual emotional turbulence, which eventually lead to her struggling with depression. Don't misunderstand me, she dressed and still to this day, dresses immaculately and is still obsessive about her cleanliness and dietary needs. Maybe it was ignorance in her peak years of health, not been told the dangers of how negative thinking could affect you in later life, that really caused her demise. But suffering a lost childhood greatly influenced the way in how she saw herself and my father's abusive behaviour added to her low self esteem. She always struggled to show us affection in the form of hugs or to say I love you. How could she understand the importance of these feelings, when she was never shown them herself from being a child. Here we are now decades later, mother has intense lower back pain with an inoperative crumbling L5 and L4 (discs) putting pressure on her sensory nerves causing weak legs leading to atrophy. Not wanting to create more pain by increased walking, she only shuffles from her lounge to her kitchen, then bathroom and bedroom. Her home has become her keeper, her prison. I needed to encourage her physical ability, refresh her body's energy, because I knew it would stimulate muscle memory as well as oxygenate her brain, which would eventually lead to a more positive healthier person. I needed to re-engage her inner child and what better way than to bounce her way back to health on a rebounder, (I checked that this was ok with her GP before going ahead and he agreed). I wanted my mother back the way I remembered her, not ravaged by old age, was that too much to ask, too greedy of me. Yes, we are all going towards that stage of life and yes my inner child is rescuing my mother, may be its me meeting my needs and not hers, maybe she doesn't want to be saved, may be as she says from time to time, she is just waiting to die, but I'm not giving her that choice. You may think it unkind and selfish of me, but another cruel twist of fate has added another condition to the list of my mother's illnesses. She has recently been diagnosed with the early stages of Dementia. I am now the responsible adult who is taking care of her, knowing what is best for my children means I have the tools now to support my mother; with respect, I will be taken her under my wings, to protect her from herself, because I know that in time, she will no longer know herself or me. For now, she enjoys the gifts that rebounding has brought her, more strength in her legs and more laughter, as she bounces her way back to health.

PROTECTING YOUR MIND

The statistics are growing at an alarming rate; more people are being diagnosed with Alzheimer's and Dementia than at any other period of time. What is it about 21st century living that is making our minds go into this black hole. Is it because we are now living longer than ever before, surely not. I believe the impact of daily stress in our lives has to be a part of it. I understand it can also be genetics, but we can't seem to get away from stress and the negative chatter we have in our mind when life becomes too stretched.

The great thing about rebounding is that it is so easy, only takes a few minutes a day and heals so much of our mind and body, more so than any other exercise we do. So why isn't everybody doing it? I believe it boils down to not giving yourself any time to do things for you, am I right or am I right! Taking some time daily to help ourselves is the biggest way to improve and heal both the adult and the inner child, our conscious and subconscious mind. Meditation and mindfulness heals and releases pressures in the brain created by stress, it allows us to eliminate worry, anxiety, fear, rejection, the greatest things humans dread the most. Then why not make time to do it. Don't complain it's difficult especially if you haven't even tried it! It's actually extremely easy, so easy that it's ridiculously funny that we still don't give ourselves permission to do it. Again this boils down to valuing ourselves. We learn about value from our childhood and our beliefs from the age of 3 to 8. It is this period of time in our life that our inner child develops the understanding of value, respect and love. This understanding whatever you learn as a child, will dominate the subconscious mind (where the inner child lives) for the rest of your adult life. Not having these needs met may create failures in future relationships, success, self esteem and self worth. We are also taught to help others before ourselves, as my mother did all her life. This conditioning of self sacrifice so prevalent in the 50's 60's 70's and also in many cultures and religions, has a guilt attachment branded in our psyche that becomes one of the main contributors to poor self worth.

If I asked you where I would find you in the 'caring' queue, let me guess- the majority of you would be at the very back. Why put yourself there, because you have been conditioned to believe it's the right place to be, serving others before yourself. We constantly do this to ourselves. Serving dinner we serve others before our self and especially when we give them the best cuts of meat and leave ourselves the scrappy bits. Pouring tea, we pour others before our self, again this is only etiquette and manners I hear you shout and yes I would agree. I am not asking you to suddenly break habits of a lifetime, but I am asking you to make small changes wherever possible by letting you go first from time to time. In primary school at playtime we are taught to take turns and when someone doesn't all hell breaks loose. We are told if an airplane suddenly spiralled out of control and the oxygen masks came down who would you put the mask on first, you or your children? The answer you so correctly thought is yourself. If you tried to put the mask on your first child, you wouldn't have time to complete the task as you would lose consciousness so you didn't help or save anyone. In this situation you must save yourself first in order to save others. It's about introducing more balance in your life so that you get regular turns too. When we meet our inner child's needs, then we are not as frustrated, angry and lost as individuals. We no longer have to blame others or circumstances for our failures and disappointments in life.

THE FACTS ABOUT REBOUNDING

The study of the human body is fascinating. The moment it becomes no less than amazing is when we understand what happens as the body is placed under the demands of movement and resistance we call exercise. For people who contact me to book an LT Therapy treatment, but struggle to come to the clinic due to excessive weight issues or mobility problems, I recommend rebounding as it is the first step forward in conquering these issues. Rebounding is an effective exercise that reduces your body fat; firms your arms, legs, thighs, abdomen, and hips; increases your agility; strengthens your muscles overall; provides an aerobic effect for your cardiopulmonary systems; rejuvenates your body when it's tired, and generally puts you in a state of mental and physical wellness. Helps combat stress and supports muscle memory.

The idea of rebounding has been around for a long time, but it gained popularity in the 1980s when NASA studied its benefits while trying to find an effective way to help astronauts recover and regain bone and muscle mass after being in space. Astronauts can lose as much as 15% of their bone and muscle mass from only 14 days at zero gravity, so NASA needed a way to help reverse this damage.

Some of the findings of the NASA study:

When the astronauts were tested while running on a treadmill, the G-force measured at the ankle was over twice what it was at the back and head. This means that the foot and leg absorb much of the force when running, which can explain the higher rates of foot, shin and knee problems from running (especially running incorrectly). On a trampoline, the G-force was almost identical at the ankle, back and head and at a lower level than that of the G-force at the ankle on a treadmill. This shows that rebounding can exercise the entire body without excess pressure to the feet and legs.

The external work output at equivalent levels of oxygen uptake were significantly greater while trampolining than running. The greatest difference was about 68%. In other words, the increased G-force in rebounding means you get more benefit with less oxygen used and less exertion on the heart.

HOW REBOUNDING WORKS

Many types of exercise are done to target specific muscles or just to increase cardiovascular function. Rebounding is unique since it uses the forces of acceleration and deceleration and can work on every cell in the body in a unique way.

When you bounce on a rebounder (mini-trampoline), several actions happen:

- An acceleration action as you bounce upward
- A split-second weightless pause at the top
- A deceleration at an increased G-force
- Impact to the rebounder
- Repeat

The action of rebounding makes use of the increased G-force from gravity based exercises like this and each cell in the body has to respond to the acceleration and deceleration. The up and down motion is beneficial for the lymphatic system since it runs in a vertical direction in the body.

REASONS TO REBOUND

- Rebounding provides an increased G-force (gravitational load), which strengthens the musculoskeletal systems.
- Rebounding protects the joints from the chronic fatigue and impact delivered by exercising on hard surfaces.

- Rebounding helps manage body composition and improves muscle-to-fat ratio. Rebounding diminishes body fat, improves muscle tone, improves the efficiency with which the body burns carbohydrate, and lowers pulse rate and blood pressure.
- Rebounding aids lymphatic circulation by stimulating the millions of one-way valves in the lymphatic system. Your lymphatic system acts as your body's internal vacuum cleaner.
- Rebounding circulates more oxygen to the tissues-and where there is oxygen there cannot be disease.
- Rebounding establishes a better equilibrium between the oxygen required by the tissues and the oxygen made available.
- Rebounding increases capacity for respiration.
- Rebounding tends to reduce the height to which the arterial pressures rise during exertion.
- Rebounding lessens the time during which blood pressure remains abnormal after severe activity.
- Rebounding assists in the rehabilitation of a heart problem.
- Rebounding increases the functional activity of the red bone marrow in the production of red blood cells.
- Rebounding improves resting metabolic rate so that more calories are burned for hours after exercise.
- Rebounding helps fluid move easily within the body, thus helping muscle performance and lightening the load required of the heart.
- Rebounding decreases the volume of blood pooling in the veins of the cardiovascular system preventing chronic edema.
- Rebounding improves circulation. It encourages collateral circulation (the formation of new branch blood vessels that distribute blood to the heart) by increasing the capillary count in the muscles and decreasing the distance between the capillaries and the target cells.
- Rebounding strengthens the heart and other muscles in the body so that they work more efficiently.

- Rebounding allows the resting heart to beat less often. Each beat becomes more powerful and sends out a greater surge of blood around the body to nourish its 60 trillion cells.
- Rebounding lowers circulating cholesterol and triglyceride levels.
- Rebounding lowers low-density lipoprotein (bad) in the blood and increases high-density lipoprotein (good) holding off the incidence of coronary artery disease.
- Rebounding promotes tissue repair.
- Rebounding for longer than 20 minutes at a moderate intensity increases the mitochondria count within the muscle cells, essential for endurance.
- Rebounding adds to the alkaline reserve of the body, which may be of significance in an emergency requiring prolonged effort.
- Rebounding improves coordination between the propreoceptors in the joints, the transmission of nerve impulses to and from the brain, transmission of nerve impulses and responsiveness of the muscle fibres.
- Rebounding improves the brain's responsiveness to the vestibular apparatus within the inner ear, thus improving balance.
- Rebounding offers relief from neck, shoulder and back pains, headaches, and other pain caused by lack of exercise.
- Rebounding enhances digestion and elimination processes.
- Rebounding allows for deeper and easier relaxation and sleep.
- Rebounding results in better mental performance, with keener learning processes.
- Rebounding curtails fatigue and menstrual discomfort for women.
- Rebounding minimizes the number of colds, allergies, digestive disturbances, and abdominal problems.
- Rebounding tends to slow down atrophy in the ageing process: Rebounding can actually reverse, prevent or diminish the hardening of the arteries. By conquering this

ultimate pathology, you will keep your mind alert, skin smooth, skeleton flexible, libido intact, kidneys functioning, blood circulating, liver detoxifying, enzyme systems alive, hold memory intact, and avoid all systems of the ageing process.

- Rebounding is an effective modality by which the user gains a sense of control and an improved self image.
- Rebounding supplies a reserve of bodily strength and physical efficiency.
- Rebounding helps the body attain peak cell function through chemical function.
- Rebounding expands the capacity for fuel storage, resulting in extra endurance.
- Rebounding stimulates metabolism. Rebounding provides for a better absorption.
- Rebounding increases the capacity for respiration. Breathing is controlled by changes in the volume of the chest cavity brought about mainly by muscular movements of the diaphragm; Repeated rebounding exercise accomplishes more muscle movements of the diaphragm with the consequent chest expansion.
- Rebounding boosts red blood cells. Rebounding increases the functional activity of the red bone marrow in the production of red blood cells. The red blood cells carry oxygen and nutrients to the tissues of the body and also help remove carbon dioxide from them.
- Rebounding helps fight fatigue. Rebounding tones the glandular system to increase the output of the thyroid gland, the pituitary gland and the adrenals-which all help to restore energy.
- Rebounding exercises every part of your body.
- Rebounding is fun and enjoyable!

People who rebound find they are able to work longer, sleep better, and feel less tense and nervous. The effect is not just psychological, because the action of bouncing up and down against gravity, without trauma to the musculoskeletal system, is one of the most beneficial aerobic exercises ever developed.

Though rebounding is a gentle activity, it is best to start with feet on the rebounder and only gentle bouncing by bending the knees, work up to jumping with feet leaving the rebounder as you grow confident.

Let rebounding be your body's daily movement, as well as stretching with a foam roller (as covered in chapter 9). If we prepare NOW to help ourselves, we can prevent long term back pain and believe you me, we WILL be fabulously heading towards a 'pain free' old age.

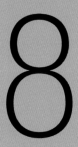

BRING ME SUNSHINE

'So much joy you can give to each brand new bright tomorrow.
Bring me fun, bring me sunshine bring me love.'

Morecambe & Wise

Who doesn't remember the fabulous comedy duo Morecambe and Wise. Growing up in the 1970's and 80's saw an abundance of brilliant comedy talent that filled our television screen, Stanley Baxter, Les Dawson, The Comedians, as well as the controversial ones such as Dave Alan and Benny Hill all broke us out in belly laughs. My favourites shows were; The Goodies, Reginald Perrin, Faulty Towers, Mash, Love Thy Neighbour, Bless This House, On the Buses, Rising Damp and Porridge. I remember laughing my way through life no matter how difficult things were and it always helped keep me focused and motivated. Fast forward to 2008, when one day my 15 year old son asked me if I had ever had a sense of humour. I paused for a moment and thought what an odd question, so I asked him what made him say that. 'It's just because I've never heard you laugh out loud or even belly laugh, as far back as I can remember.' That comment stuck with me for years as I started to look back and examine why I had stopped laughing. Then it dawned on me-I got married. From the age of 21, I stepped up and took responsibility into running a home, fulltime job and committing to all the things grown up's do. May be my inner child wasn't as ready as I thought for this sort of responsibility. What is it about turning 20 and seeking independence, is it a sign of 'look at me I've made it.' Maybe I was naive thinking I had conquered the world with a house purchase and kitting it out in Laura Ashley. I think the youth of today do that same sort of thing, to get love, connection and recognition from their peer group. They can't do it on the property ladder as I did it, it was difficult, but easier back then, than it is now, they now have Facebook to load up with selfie pictures, posting odd pouting poses and extreme face pulling. Not one to criticise, maybe this new generation is one that is reluctant to let go of childhood and still be one in the form of an adult. Girls in particular apply Barbie doll hair extensions, long acrylic talons, large hooped earrings, 6" killer heels, botox, fillers, semi permanent make up, cosmetic lifts and enhancements, finishing off with a permanent 'orange' tan. Driven to seek solace in alcohol, binge drinking with friends, jager bombs, what is the message they are sending out to the world. Possibly a lost youth, their inner child still searching for love.

LAUGHTER IS THE BEST MEDICINE

They say that laughter is the best medicine to healing all emotional and physical pain. You've heard of people making miraculous recoveries from tumours the size of grapefruits simply through laughing their way back to health, so let's bring more of it into our lives. Oh you already do, well you may think you do as I did, but in today's crazy, busy world, keeping a sense of humour is vital. Most of the clients I see in clinic are so down and stressed because of their back pain whether chronic or acute, they soon forget to laugh because as they say, there's now't much to laugh about.

During the two World Wars Britain was strong in keeping a

stiff upper lip, embracing as much laughter in such dark times. They made a real effort to squeeze happy moments in a perilous period. With food so scarce due to heavy rationing, having a laugh was a healthy way to keep positive. One of the best feelings in the world is the deep-rooted belly laugh. It can bring people together and establish amazing connections. Everything from a slight giggle to a side-splitting stitch can change the temperature of a room from chilly unfamiliarity to a warm family-like atmosphere. There is so much to love about laughter that it seems greedy to look for more, but that's exactly what researchers at the Loma Linda University in California did finding some amazing results.

Laughing lowers blood pressure - People who lower their blood pressure even those who start at normal levels, will reduce their risk of strokes and heart attacks

Reduces stress hormone levels - You benefit from reducing the level of stress hormones your body produces because hormone-level reduction simultaneously cuts the anxiety and stress impacting your body. Additionally, the reduction of stress hormones in your body may result in higher immune system performance. Just think: Laughing along as a co-worker tells a funny joke can relieve some of the day's stress and help you reap the health benefits of laughter.

Fun workout - One of the benefits of laughter is that it can help you tone your body. When you are laughing, the muscles in your stomach expand and contract, similar to when you intentionally exercise your abs. Meanwhile, the muscles you are not using to laugh are getting an opportunity to relax. Gives a workout to the diaphragm and abdominal, respiratory, facial, leg, and back muscles.

Improves cardiac health - Laughter is a great cardio workout, especially for those who are incapable of doing other physical activity due to injury or illness. It gets your heart pumping and burns a similar amount of calories per hour as walking at a slow to moderate pace. Increase vascular blood flow and oxygenation of the blood

Improve your immune system - Negative thoughts manifest into chemical reactions that can affect your body by bringing more stress into your system and decreasing your immunity. In contrast, positive thoughts and laughter actually release neuropeptides that help fight stress and potentially more-serious illnesses. Laughing defends against respiratory infections—even reducing the frequency of colds—by immunoglobulin in saliva.

Triggers the release of endorphins - Endorphins are the body's natural pain killers. By laughing, you can release endorphins, which can help ease chronic pain and make you feel good all over. Laughter may also break the pain-spasm cycle common to some muscle disorders.

Produces a general sense of well-being - Laughter can increase your overall sense of well-being. Doctors have found that people who have a positive outlook on life tend to fight diseases better than people who tend to be more negative. Increases memory and learning; in a study at Johns Hopkins University Medical School, humour during instruction led to increased test scores. Improve alertness, creativity, and memory.

Humour works quickly. Less than a half-second after exposure to something funny, electrical waves move through the higher brain functions of the cerebral cortex. The left hemisphere analyses the words and structures of the joke; the right hemisphere "gets" the joke; the visual sensory area of the occipital lobe creates images; the limbic (emotional) system makes you happier; and the motor sections make you smile or laugh. Simple isn't it. The next time you feel down, suffer chronic back pain, put on a great comedy show or film. The classics of Charlie Chaplin, Laurel & Hardy, The Marx Brothers and Norman Wisdom will have you in stitches in no time. With the latest mobile phone screens and ipads you can be sat on the train enjoying such moments, who needs a TV!

JEAN'S STORY

We tend to take for granted each day we have and those who share it with us, due to all the running around and routine ruts we bury ourselves in. Jean was a busy housewife, mother and grandmother who had been happily married to Paul for over 30 years. Paul was a businessman and experienced cyclist, who had cycled most of his life. Jean remembers that spring morning in May 2014 well. It was the day Paul was leaving to start the Yorkshire Tour De France route with two of his best friends. They were doing the route before the actual Tour came to Yorkshire in the July. The men were excited like little school boys getting ready for a go-cart race. Well equipped and fully prepared, Jean reflected on what she would do with herself that weekend, the house would be empty, as both children now lived with their partners. She gave Paul a big squeeze, as he kissed her cheek a cold shiver went down her spine. She gazed into his eyes and he was gone. That was the last time Jean would see Paul alive. Sunday came and so did an unexpected call. Rushing to answer the phone Jean expecting to hear Paul's voice updating her with how the ride was going. It was his best friend telling her that Paul had suffered a major fatal heart attack whilst riding and collapsed at the road side. The Yorkshire Air Ambulance crew had arrived within minutes whilst CPR was being performed, but the medics said he died instantly. The days that followed were a daze for Jean her world had caved in, Paul was her rock and now he was gone. She was so dependent on him in every way; she was left now picking up the pieces.

She came to see me in the July suffering severe neck and shoulder pains. It had begun to affect her arms and lower back, she felt a right mess. She told me how she had heard about my work the year before and made a mental note to pay a visit as she had back problems on and off over the past 12 years.

After Paul's death they got worse, she read an article in the local press about my LT Therapy work and decided it was time to sort herself out. Prior to the treatment, I knew nothing about Paul or his sudden passing. As I began working on her tight shoulders I spoke about an upset with her daughter, son and grandson, I then went onto her left side of the neck where her husband's energy would be and it was solid, as hard a stone, equally her right side was too. I explained that this would relate to difficulties in her relationship or sudden loss or bereavement. Jean burst into tears and told me all about the unexpected changes in her world through his death. She had to organise all the finances, home, sort through his things and decide her own future. The treatment released 90% of her tightness as muscle memory was reset. In her homecare advice sheet, I asked her to think about what she wanted to do for herself without attaching guilt. It had been three months since Paul's death and she hadn't stopped to think about her needs once. Her lower back pain was her inner child feeling vulnerable; her shoulders were her worries for how her children and grandson was coping with the shock of the loss. I asked her to put herself first and focus on her life or she would struggle to improve both mentally and physically. She had always wanted to set her own business up as a Reflexologist after training in the discipline five years earlier, but never progressed further. She had a love for sailing, but never had a chance to learn it. By the time I saw her two weeks later at her review there was a different Jean that walked through my door. She glowed with delight at having for the first time a pain free neck and shoulders, the flexibility had been restored and she felt a weight lifted from her entire back. She told me that she struggled for a few days after the treatment as her muscles adjusted to the release, but then she felt great within herself. She started to sleep better which made it easier for her to make clearer decisions about the way forward. She designed a new business card and set up as a freelance mobile reflexologist. I couldn't believe her amazing transformation and there was more. She signed up to do a six week sailing course at the local lake which brought Jean's smile back. I went on to treat her son and daughter successfully. Jean continues to thrive almost a year after her husband's death. Her family have raised lots of money for the Yorkshire Air Ambulance in memory of Paul. Jean learnt to smile and laugh again after such a great loss. She looked ahead and listened to what her mind and body needed, she did not suffer in silence like so many of us do. There isn't a day that goes by that Jean doesn't miss or think of Paul, but she laughs with joy at the good times they had together and feels by doing this she is continually healing herself.

LIFTING YOUR MOOD

Pain provokes an emotional response in everyone. If you have pain, you may also have high anxiety, irritability, and agitation. These are very normal feelings when you're hurting. Normally, as pain subsides, so does the stressful response. But with chronic pain, you may feel constantly tense and stressed. Over time, the constant stress can result in different emotional problems associated with low mood and depression.

Some of the overlap between depression and chronic pain can be explained by biology. Depression and chronic pain share some of the same neurotransmitters – brain chemicals that act as messengers travelling between nerves. Depression and chronic pain also share some of the same nerve pathways. The impact of chronic pain on a person's life also contributes to depression. Chronic pain can force you to struggle with tremendous losses, such as the loss of exercise, sleep, social network, relationships, sexual relationships, even a job and income. These losses can make you feel depressed. Depression then magnifies the pain and reduces your coping skills. While you used to exercise and be active when you felt stressed, with chronic pain you can no longer deal with stress in this manner. Because chronic pain and depression are so intertwined, they are often treated together. Many people with chronic pain avoid exercise. But, if you don't exercise, you get out of shape and have an increased risk of injury and worsened pain. Consult with your doctor to design an exercise plan that's safe and effective for you. Exercise also helps ease depression by releasing the same kind of brain chemicals that antidepressant medications release. So for those people who want to avoid tablets, exercise is Mother Nature's way of healing your pain.

Back pain affects your ability to live, work, and play the way you're used to. This can change how you see yourself sometimes for the worse as you feel victimised by the pain and low mood. To help lift your mood you need to change your focus and learn to become more optimistic. Try to consider the sunny side of a situation rather than focusing on the negative. If it's pouring rain, think of the good it will do for your garden. Fake it and you'll feel sunnier. In a Clark University study, one group of participants was told to smile and another group was told to frown. Afterward, both groups were shown cartoons and the smilers rated the shows funnier than the frowners did. The simple act of smiling seems to activate happiness centres in the brain, reports lead researcher James Laird, PhD. A University of Missouri–Columbia study says stroking a dog for just 15 minutes releases the feel-good hormones serotonin, prolactin, and oxytocin, and lowers the stress hormone cortisol and if you're more of a cat person? No worries: Other research has found that playing with your kitty gives a similar mood and health boost.

Feeling stressed and overwhelmed is a common trigger for low mood symptoms and neck, shoulder back pain. If you're struggling with pain, it's important not to over schedule your time and take on more than you can manage. If you have complicated tasks to perform at work or at home, break them up into manageable pieces. And remember: It's OK to slow down a bit. What you eat affects your brain, not just your body, so if you're feeling low, it's important to eat a healthy, balanced diet rich in whole grains, fruits, vegetables, and protein. Some foods may affect your mood more than others. For example, carbohydrates and foods that contain vitamin D boost levels of serotonin, a neurotransmitter associated with mood and some research suggests that omega-3 fatty acids, which are found in fish and fish-oil supplements, can help fight depression and pain.

DEBBIE'S STORY

Debbie came to my clinic with poor mobility in her upper back, shoulder and neck muscles. She was a 44 year old mother of two who had been on a rollercoaster journey with her struggle to cope with severe panic attacks. You couldn't wish to meet a lovelier lady than Debbie, she was Mary Poppins without the umbrella, always helping others and most definitely putting herself last. Her panic attacks were increasing rapidly to the point she was barely venturing out to do normal tasks like the school run, shopping and work. She took two attempts to get to me and I was surprised to see she arrived so calm, but I could spot the signs being a reformed sufferer. After the usual medical consultation, I started to work on her most blocked areas in the upper back which all related to past relationship, family and work. Her SCM muscle which dominates the neck and attaches to the clavicle bone at the front of the chest was the tightest I had seen for a long time; this was one of the areas that was triggering her panic attacks. She was secretly clenching her jaw adding more tension to the muscle and heightening her anxiety. Things had started to spiral out of control as Debbie was coming to the end of a bitter divorce after discovering her husband was seeing another woman. The shock that ended what she thought was the 'perfect' marriage was soul destroying for her as she struggled to come to terms with the deceit. Debbie had a very strong supportive loving family, but even with this, it was her own inner child battling with her poor self esteem since childhood that was sabotaging her adult mind, throwing her body into complete disarray. Her Yin and Yang energy was unbalanced and she felt this lack of control through her constant daily attacks. She had little reserves to fight back. I identified that as she found it difficult to accept this deception, her panic attacks would continue. She had to start working to accept what had happened, move herself to the front of the queue and acknowledge her inner child. I wasn't asking Debbie to rebuild her childhood foundations, they were strong, it was rebuilding her adult self esteem that was needed to slow down her attacks. She had to learn to take control of herself and see the rejection as a time to grow. I gave Debbie a few things to be working on for home care (as shown in Chapter 9) and reviewed her back a week later. What a difference seven days make, she had improved mobility by 90% to her neck and shoulder muscles and cut her panic attacks from ten a day to three. She started to learn what to watch for, what triggered them. She kept a diary and wrote her emotional mood down. If she had a worse day with the attacks, she looked back in her diary to see how she felt the day before. Slowly over two months and seeing Debbie every two weeks, she took control and stopped suffering from both anxiety and panic attacks. She learned to spot the signs that would generate an attack and took steps to prevent it happening. She felt liberated to be herself again and enjoyed the freedom of living life to the full.

Understanding the importance of smiling, laughing and keeping positive no matter how dark and difficult times can get is another natural way to heal you physical pain. Legendary actor Tim Curry, who suffered a devastating stroke in 2012 at the age of 67, said having a sense of humour was vital to his recovery. If you are suffering a problematic life, don't feel that your mood has to fit the situation. If life gets you down and everyone around you is pessimistic, then you don't have to be the same. Judge the situation and allow yourself to smile, don't feel guilty just because everyone else is miserable. Move yourself to the front of the 'care giving' queue and do what suits you in order to preserve you and allow healing to begin inside and out.

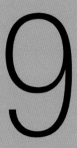

9

'AIN'T NO MOUNTAIN HIGH ENOUGH'

'My love is alive way down in my heart although we are miles apart'

Sung by Marvin Gaye & Tammi Terrell

I want you jumping around the room, singing and shaking to the beat of this song. Not because it's the last chapter of my self help book, but because I want you to do something out of the ordinary, I want you to break protocol and see what it feels like to do an unscheduled task. If you don't know the tune, then download it onto your phone or play it back through your computer. It's three minutes of telling yourself 'I can do it' 'I am in control' and like the song says' ain't no mountain high enough.' Once again interpretation is in the ear of the beholder and I, listening to this tune am singing to all the three people in me, parent, adult and inner child. I am learning to reconnect with myself. The joy music gives us is so self healing within the depths of our soul, it is releasing our darkest demons to reinstate a euphoric feeling that consumes our whole being. Appreciating and valuing what we have daily in our lives is the essence of true happiness. Taking for granted our family, friends, loved ones and what we already have is our downfall. Eventually it will lead to our physical pain and a world trapped in self pity.

When we are young, we can't wait to get old and when we get old, we want to be young again. Why can't we just love living in the time we are in, why do we become so disillusioned, is it pressure of responsibility, work, building relationships, forming friendships, maintaining our status in society, keeping up appearances, its all of these and more. As humans we need to grow inside ourselves. We need to feel fulfilled as individuals, in order to achieve this we have to have good foundations to begin with or at least the belief that we can make it strong. If you build your own home, would you succeed if the foundations were made of straw? No, you'd ensure you use reinforced concrete so those foundations would be there long after you left this planet. My foundations were rocky to start with, but I used those humble beginnings as a template to better myself, I'm sure you know of many famous people who became extraordinary through a difficult childhood. When we don't grow and everyone else around us seems to overtake us, we begin to feel sorry for ourselves. Self pity is a useless emotion that we need to flush away. A good portion of people reading this will ignore what I just wrote and continue to feel sorry for themselves. They'll tell themselves that they're **different**, that they have it **worse than everyone else**, and that **no one understands** what they're going through.

The truth is that people feel sorry for themselves because it **feels good** to feel sorry for yourself. Self pity is comforting, because it allows us to **blame external forces for our misfortunes**. It justifies not taking action when taking action would be difficult, stressful, and where it could lead to failure. Self pity brings emotional and physical pain.

Is there someone in your life who seems to always feel sorry for him or herself? Do you find yourself offering advice that never gets accepted? And do you feel guilty, because instead of sympathising with their difficulties, you frequently feel frustrated with them? Let's be clear here. Most of us are totally sympathetic with friends, family members, co-workers and even acquaintances when they feel sorry for themselves on occasion, whether the reason seems big or even almost insignificant. We are also ready to intervene, if we can, to protect someone who is being hurt or abused by someone stronger or more powerful. What we are talking about here is someone who feels sorry for them self almost all of the time, and who wants us to join in his/her self-pity.

So what makes someone feel sorry for themselves all (or a lot) of the time? And what makes it so hard for us to feel genuine sympathy for them?

Often it seems people who feel like this are really looking for help, but really that's the last thing they want. This need to have our feelings recognised is sometimes called a need for "mirroring." Peter Fonagy, a British psychologist, is one of a number of people who have been looking at the importance of mirroring from others. According to him, in order to know what we feel, we need someone else to reflect our emotions back to us. Another way to put this is that we need to have our feelings validated by others.

Unfortunately, people who feel sorry for themselves on a regular basis often have the opposite experience. Other people try to get them to look on the bright side of things instead of validating or affirming their internal pain. So they reject the advice and continue to dwell on their own suffering, and people get irritated with them instead of feeling sympathetic. This becomes a vicious cycle that is very difficult to get out of. If you find it hard to be genuinely sympathetic with someone who regularly sees themselves as a victim, you're in good company. We tend to be more readily sympathetic towards someone who we consider mentally strong, who has had an unfortunate experience and is trying to move on from it. Mentally strong people don't "waste time feeling sorry for them self." Most of us admire this trait and hope that we can be considered in that group ourselves. So it can be hard to empathise with someone who seems unwilling to try to get them self into a better place They may reject all suggestions that would help them. They may seem to get more pleasure from complaining than from trying to improve things. No matter how desperate a person longs to have their pain recognised, they may also unconsciously feel that they deserve to suffer. This is not usually something they recognise or can communicate to others. They may even genuinely appreciate it when someone recognises how much they are suffering. But because they feel guilty or undeserving of that recognition, they need to reject it. What often seems even worse is that the person who looks at life through a negative lens never acknowledges when good things happen to them, or when they actually seem to have a stroke of good luck. What can you do to help yourself if you feel like this or deal with a person in your own life that suffers the same?

Understanding -Sometimes it helps simply to understand, as we have just tried to do, something about how self-pity works.

Sympathise - I have found that while a simple expression of sympathy can sometimes help, it is often not enough to stop the onslaught of feelings. But it can help to give a more expressive, emotional response, like, "Oh, that sounds so terrible. You must really be suffering! I'm so sorry to hear about it.'

Advice - If you must give advice, do it with the awareness that it will probably not be accepted, and if it is accepted, it will probably not be followed through. Knowing ahead of time that there are reasons that the best of advice may not work for this person in your life can help you feel less frustrated by their behaviour.

Recognition - It's useful to recognise not only the pain, but the feelings of helplessness and frailty that this person may feel. Although help rejecting complainers may appear strong, they may be much more vulnerable than they seem. It's not easy, but if you can acknowledge both their strengths and their sense of being mistreated, sometimes that really can help them move forward.

SURE, BAD THINGS HAPPEN

Obviously not everything that happens to us is within our control. Accidents happen, people die, illness can strike, and fate can be cruel. But no matter what happens, **you and you alone** get to play the cards you're dealt. You get to choose how you react when you lose your job, when you relapse and end up in rehab again, when your significant other cheats on you with your best friend.

STOP FOCUSING ON WHAT OTHER PEOPLE HAVE

The more you focus on what other people have and what you don't, the more you're going to feel sorry for yourself. The more you feel sorry for yourself, the less you're going to move forward in your life. Despite what you might tell yourself, I can **guarantee** that not everyone who has it better than you, started out with less than you. There are also people in this world who were born with a silver spoon. They've had everything handed to them without having to work for it. They might even be arrogant about it, even though they did nothing to deserve their good fortune.

You know what? Be happy for them. Why not? How does their good fortune affect your life in anyway? You only get to play the hand you're dealt, and the more energy you spend obsessing over someone else's lot in life, the less energy you'll have to work towards improving your own.

As I mentioned earlier, one of the reasons it's so hard to get rid of self pity is because it's such a comforting emotion. It doesn't take any effort to feel sorry for yourself, but it takes tremendous effort to overcome life's challenges and become a better person for it.

To make things worse, once self pity sets in, **it becomes an**

ingrained pattern in our mind that's hard to get rid of. We get trained to think negatively, to start the pity party when things don't go well for us. So what can you do the next time you start feeling sorry for yourself?

1. Implement a Zero tolerance policy

Start by telling yourself that you are no longer going to feel sorry for yourself. Right now, stop reading and take a moment to make this commitment to yourself.

It's not going to be easy; you have ingrained patterns in your brain that encourage self-pity. But the next two steps should help you slowly but surely create new patterns.

2. Build Self Esteem

Self-esteem can be a wonderful tool for fighting off self-pity. When you feel strong and confident in yourself, you have little need to feel sorry for yourself. Of course, building self-esteem is not an easy thing to do, especially if you're used to self-loathing and pity.

Building true self-esteem is a process that you work on bit by bit, day by day. Here are some things you can do to improve your sense of self-worth:

- Exercise regularly and get into great shape
- Learn about nutrition and start eating healthy
- Do charity work
- Meditate
- Form new hobbies that requires socialising
- Do new things that are out of your comfort zone
- Set small goals for yourself. Use these stepping stones to work towards achieving bigger goals.
- Learn solid financial management. Learn that you don't need to spend money to be happy, and that the things you own don't define your worth, this for me is extremely important and so very true.

Don't expect overnight changes, because they won't happen. But if you keep striving for a tiny bit of personal improvement each day, one day you'll look back at your old self and marvel at how much you've changed. These small steps daily will add up to big changes and going in the positive direction is a step closer to resolving your pain.

3. Be grateful for what you have

Is the glass half full or half empty? Even if the glass is only 1/100 full, the way we choose to perceive it is the thing that counts.

No matter how little you have, there's no doubt you have things to be grateful for. The fact that you have access to the internet right now, connected to the world's information superhighway and reading the thoughts of another human being thousands of miles away is a miracle in itself.

Choosing to be grateful for what you have is a direct attack on self pity. You can't be grateful and feel sorry for yourself at the same time. Of course, if you're used to choosing self-pity, it might be difficult to get into a grateful mindset.

To retrain your negative thought patterns, I want you to try this exercise. Every single day for the next month, write down 5 things you're grateful for every morning. Do it without fail.

It can be as simple as being thankful for the fresh morning air, that first sip of hot coffee in the morning, the smell of fresh bacon in the frying pan, or even the fact that you're alive. You can repeat the same 5 things everyday if you want, as long as you take the time to come up with 5 reasons to be grateful and write them down. Daily repetition in being grateful for these things no matter how small will help the mind refocus on a more positive outlook. Self-pity is a habit and a choice. Take actions to unlearn this negative habit, and choose to bring some positivity into your life.

DENISE'S STORY

I saw Denise at my Harley Street Clinic in London, she had suffered from problems in her back, neck and shoulders for years. She had been to see endless chiropractors and physiotherapists, but every treatment was only temporary. Then a friend recommended she see me after reading about my work in a health magazine. I clearly remember when I first saw her, how tired and exhausted she looked, ravaged by pain that had reduced her to being a very negative and sceptical person pre-judging everything including my treatment. After the usual general health questionnaire Denise lay on the couch and I began to trace through her timeline why her muscles were so tight. Using the heat and ice to transcend into the muscle and reset muscle memory, her tightest side was the left, male energy. I could feel within her energy that she had had a long ongoing battle with a male and suggested it may be an ex-husband. She confirmed that she had gone through a very stressful divorce that had dragged on for over eight years. Denise thought she had put it behind her, yes literally it was physically holding on to her back muscles, controlled by her subconscious mind. She had low self esteem and was filled with feeling sorry for herself, a result of a long difficult marriage. As I worked through the blocked areas, Denise felt a sudden deep sadness which made her become very tearful, this I explained was part of the process and I encouraged her to not hold back. She felt an incredible sense of relief. When I reviewed her neck shoulders and back four weeks later to check how her muscle memory had held, I barely recognised the person who walked through my door. Denise looked simply amazing; with a twinkle in her eyes and peachy skin I thought she had been to a studio for a makeover. She laughed out loud when I told her, even though she was a part time model, she had not had anything of the kind for years. The day she left the clinic, she slept so well and deeply, her journey of self discovery and recovery began. She felt a renewed energy within her. It triggered her to start doing all the things she always wanted to but felt held back. She put her house on the market and sold it within a week; she found her dream home in the same week and won a lucrative modelling contract she had never dreamed she was good enough to get. When you believe in yourself and acknowledge your inner child, you have found the essence of who you truly are, anything and everything is possible. After those two treatments I didn't need to see Denise again. She still keeps in touch to tell me how great her back feels and now when she gets any niggles, it's her back telling her to do more exercise not negative emotional pain from her inner child.

LT RECOVERY GUIDE

The following tips are tried and tested proven techniques to help kick start your journey of recovery from back pain and at the same time help you discover your inner child, the real you. It shows you how to start focusing and developing to bring more balance into your life, leading to the true you.(Remember if you have any medical conditions or regular prescriptive medicines, please check with your GP before participating in any of these changes.).

1. Build boundaries

Visualise a garden with a fence on four sides. Whatever you want to grow in it you can it is limitless- flowers or vegetables or both. Design how it looks, set the scene/layout, fill your garden with colour. You then decide who visits the garden or not. This is an analogy of you (you are the garden and the flowers you grow is your inner child) with this in mind every day set out what your day will be like; appointments, free time to do what you like such as shopping, cooking, baking, sewing, knitting, painting, dancing, walking, etc. Releasing creative energy is a huge part of understanding and developing ourselves it is allowing the inner child 'playtime.' So many of us do not make time for this and it is an extremely important element for balance and well being in the mind and body.

If your planned day (in your garden) is unexpectedly interrupted, you decide (as you stand in your garden by the fence) whether to allow interruption and change to affect your day, to accommodate the other person. If you want to complete what you started that day, then you have to tell the person you cannot help at that given moment but will schedule a time when you can(either later in the day or the next day etc)

By taking control of the day, unexpected events and people no longer take control of you. If you do not control your situation, you are allowing people and events to knock your fence down and take whatever they like from your garden, in most cases destroying it.

All your hard work will have been for nothing and you are left disappointed, angry, resentful, hurt and betrayed. All negative responses that if allowed to continue, create our emotional and physical pain. That's why setting boundaries is so important in our daily life.

2. Healthy Eating

What you feed the body affects your mind. The mind when happy releases dopamine and serotonin which are natural pain relief & healers in our body. When we feel positive we eat and drink healthily when we feel down depressed and negative we release adrenaline and cortisol which means we crave more processed, sugary foods and drinks such as pop and alcohol to satisfy our sad mood. We associate foods such as chocolate, cake and biscuits with comfort, willing it to make us feel better. If this state of mind continues then an unbalanced and unhealthy lifestyle ensues which can eventually lead to weight issues as well as a depressive outlook. Juicing helps support a healthy lifestyle visit www.juicemaster.com for ideas on how to add a juice a day to your diet, learn about its benefits and reap the riches of what it can do for your well being.

3. Supplements

The question is to add supplements to your diet or not? Even if you believe you have the right balance in your diet with nuts, seeds, green vegetables and oily fish it's never enough according to medical research. The older we get the quicker our system gets depleted due to environmental changes and genetic scavengers. Stress is one of those scavengers that strips our mind and body of energy, creates lethargy and a negative outlook. What can supplementing our diet do for us? Re-balance any deficiency; you'll notice you won't ache as much or at all. You'll have more energy to do things which breeds a positive outlook. Your concentration will improve. What supplements are right for you? A good one a day multivitamin. Vitabiotic is a range of vitamins well researched and created to suit today's busy lifestyles. High strength formula Omega 3 such as Efamol Omega 3 Brain Formula has added Evening Primrose oil and is an excellent choice. High strength Omega 3 supports collagen so is great for skin and joints it also supports brain cells and has been known to hold back Dementia and Alzheimer's. So if you had to supplement add a good one a day multi vitamin as well as good high strength Omega 3. Always available online or from your local pharmacy. (Certain supplements can interfere with certain medication. If you are taking any check with your GP)

4. Move More

Most people have regular exercise or classes they attend weekly. Regardless of your build, it is important to move daily as too much of a sedentary life creates mood imbalance. Some people are sedentary because of their job sitting long hours at the computer or desk concentrating on targeted deadlines, whether its sales, admin, studies or media it breeds the same result, over production of adrenaline and cortisol.

By adding more movement in your day you are ensuring the body keeps active, burns calories disperses lactic acid build up and visually changes the scenery for the brain to activate happy hormones.

Walking just 1 mile a day will help the body maintain a healthy weight, strengthen joints and muscles, physical balance and most of all change the visuals-your focus. Purchasing a cheap basic pedometer for a couple of pounds will ensure you do the minimum daily 10,000 steps as suggested by the National Health Board. Seeing something visual will encourage you to see that you are doing this and make you feel more positive, that you are going in the right direction to supporting your needs. Stretching daily will also help reduce lactic build up so before you get out of bed stretch, do regularly simple stretches during the day when it suits you and after a long stint at the desk especially.

5. Foam Roller

As we start to age our body starts to change. We need to stay injury and pain free. Whether you train regularly, do a desk job or are sedentary for long periods of time, your muscles will be prone to repetitive injury as you are straining the same muscles daily using poor posture. High intensity training impacts the body in the same way, as the person training uses the same muscles to do the same workout. Microscopic tears in the muscle are a natural occurrence when we train, but over time this leads to trigger points. These are hyper irritable points in the muscle known as knots. When you press on a trigger point it is tender and sore. A trigger point has a referral spot, for example you can press in your shoulder and feel pain in the head. Leaving trigger points (knots) untreated can lead to scar tissue in the muscle which will decrease strength, reduce flexibility and limit mobility. The other muscles in your body will then be forced to compensate for this loss and they in turn will start to form trigger points and so this vicious cycle continues. The body is a connected chain so what happens in one part will affect another. How to prevent trigger points (knots):

Ideally a sports massage, physiotherapy one session per week, but this can be very expensive. A foam roller is a simple, easy, inexpensive and effective way to release your tight muscles.

This is excellent for reducing pain throughout the whole back, glutes & legs. It can be purchased online or on the high street and sports shops. Comes with easy instructions and there are free You Tube short videos from personal trainers that show you how in a few minutes a day you can begin to have soft, flexible muscles. As always use sensibly and according to your condition, start gently and slowly build your usage up. Five/ten minutes in the morning and evening. There are two types; one with a smooth surface and one which has indentations. The one that is irregular will apply more pressure on the muscles, so if you are very inflamed and tight you're best starting off with a smooth foam roller. Ultimately your aim is to end with the 'teeth' like roller as it covers more myofascial and trigger point release work. Never roll over bone only muscle. It will feel very uncomfortable at first especially over your bottom muscles and IT bands on the side of the legs and thighs, but this will ease with regular use. Long term outcome is healthy muscles and minimum injury.

6.Sing/Dance

Adding music daily in your life will break your negative thought pattern. Choose songs that make you feel good and remind you of very happy times, this will ensure you mentally feel positive. Music and movies are our escapism and inspiration; they allow us to believe in a world of hope. William Shakespeare said;

'If music be the food of love, play on' from Twelfth Night

Songs give us hope, bring peace, uplift our spirits and make us feel good about ourselves. I know there are songs and music that do the opposite as well, but as life brings us so many daily challenges, focus on the songs that make us feel good and heal our souls. At the beginning of each chapter I take a quote from a song or film that is fun and inspirational, if you are not already doing it you need to get in touch with your music and movies. The ones you grew up with that motivate and move you that create goose bumps at the back of your neck and that make you belly laugh. Reconnect with your inner child and spirited playfulness. I was never able to watch films at the cinema when I was young; it was a luxury my parents could not afford. The only two films my father took us to see were 'Jaws' when I was 12 and 'Close Encounters of the Third Kind' when I was 14. Regardless of the genre I fell in love with the movies. I started watching the Oscars from aged 10 on TV and loved the glamour and the prestige of these events. I let my imagination run away with itself and saw myself walking up the red carpet looking as glamorous as the rest. I still have that dream today, I never doubt it won't happen, as they say, watch this space. University of Manchester researchers discovered that an organ in the inner ear (that responds to singing sounds) is connected to a part of the brain that registers pleasure. So singing, alone in the car, or in a crowd at church (even if you're very, very bad at it), may make you happier.

7. Learn Meditation

Simple easy meditation twice a day helps the mind de-stress, clears out the unnecessary negative emotions such as guilt that we hang onto, allowing our brain to re-charge itself and start a fresh. Transcendental meditation is a worldwide therapy and has the most scientific supportive evidence. Check out www.tm.org for more information. Meditation is the daily mental exercise our brains need in order to cope with challenging events, jobs, people that we face on a regular basis. By inviting it into your daily routine, you won't suffer the consequences that go with being out of control, allowing fear to dominate your mind and a negative mood.

The above can be introduced in your own pace and time, it's not a race to do it all and tick the boxes. The main thing is to take small steps equal big changes. Introduce each improvement and ensure you do it daily, repetition daily is so important. By doing these actions daily you retrain your mind and body.

TO RE-CAP - DAILY THINGS TO DO;

- Stretch
- Move more
- Sing/dance
- Healthy eating
- Drink water
- Supplements
- Laugh more
- Meditation
- Most importantly - build your boundaries towards a more balanced life

FINAL WORD

GREATEST LOVE OF ALL

'The greatest love of all is easy to achieve,
learning to love yourself it is the greatest love of all.'
Sung by Whitney Houston

Beautiful words taken from a love song but really, all love songs are primarily for our self, before others. This book has been about a journey of self discovery, of learning why it is important to love yourself before all others. When you understand and appreciate the parent, adult and inner child within you, you can heal emotionally and physical back pain will only exist because of physical trauma, instead of both. If you ignore the essence of who you really are, you are really undervaluing and burying the real you. When we silence our inner child, we are rejecting our true self. We become dysfunctional, unfulfilled individuals that follow the road to self pity, regrets and taking for granted the most important people in our lives.

'I now come to believe my past failures and frustrations were actually laying the foundation for the understandings that have created the new level of living I now enjoy.' Tony Robbins American self help author.

Tony Robbins encapsulates in words what every human suffers-failure and frustration. Whether from childhood or in adult life, we can look at these in two different ways, positive or negative. When you appreciate and acknowledge your challenges, no matter how painful, you allow yourself, the adult and inner child to grow. You value, respect and love yourself more for making the decision, taking action, rather than ignoring the person or matter .This is a healthy way to approach challenges, they are our lessons in life. Those that choose the negative option, allow their fear to control their life, seeing failure as their comfort blanket. They trap it and wrap it around their shoulders owing it for years. Repeated negative emotional patterns, produce physical pain due to muscle memory. Depending on the who, what and why, we allow it be stored in our body. All the organs, tissues and cells in the body have an energetic frequency. Negative emotions and negative thoughts have a different energetic frequency than healthy cells and tissue. Because of that, they can distort the organs, tissues and cells that surround where they are stored in the body. They become trapped in our back muscles and eventually physical pain is the result.

When the energetic frequency of the body gets too low, dis-ease has a perfect environment to live in as well as back pain. So simply put, you can improve your health by making your body an environment where dis-ease can't thrive. You do this by acknowledging the importance of giving yourself permission to 'play' through a pastime, hobby or relaxation. Allowing yourself to feel 'guilt free' instead of feeling the need to be always serving others, whether at home, work or socially.

Releasing trapped negative emotions held in the neck, shoulder and back muscles by resetting muscle memory, is the best way I know how to start letting the body self heal. Releasing trapped negative emotions can never hurt, so you have nothing to lose, its emotional baggage you didn't want anyway, right?

How many times have you told yourself it is "ridiculous to get upset over this!" or "it's not worth upsetting dad" to bring up. Those types of situations cause you to be at risk for trapping emotions, suppressing your inner child. Emotions want a "voice" and if they are not acknowledged, they won't go away. When we are isolated while dealing with a stressful event, we are at risk of trapped emotions. I believe this is because it is human nature to find comfort in the sharing of our emotions — positive and negative. When we can't reach out, we may be less likely to really feel them and experience them. It often feels safer to let go emotionally with someone else. Not having any coping skills for the specific event that's bringing up negative emotions can really leave us "stuck." If for instance it's the first time you experience something, such as the death of a loved one, you are more likely to "freeze" emotionally than you would be if you had coping skills for the situation. You would be more likely to have coping skills if you learned them during an earlier similar life event.

The top 10 negative emotions on my list are the ones I see most often, in most people. These create neck, shoulder, back pain as the emotion is held in the muscles stored through muscle memory. Now remember, these are just the ones that I commonly find to be lodged in the body. Certain events or years of your life can create different types of emotions, and even multiples of the same ones. These are just a general list of what comes up most during my treatments with clients. Also keep in mind, they don't all have to get stuck! Negative emotions aren't bad. They can only harm if you don't let them go and keep them on the repeat loop.

1. Anxiety

A general feeling of uneasiness; a fear of the unknown; fear without a subject reason.

Anxiety is probably the thing I see that most people repress. It's my belief that anxiety is just another emotion (or a mix of them) trying to come up! People can have a hard time identifying where the anxiety is coming from, what it is and when it started. It often becomes such a common feeling that we come up with all kinds of ways to ignore it.

2. Disgust

A feeling of loathing; when good taste or moral sense is offended; a strong aversion.

Disgust is a feeling that is low enough on the radar to not say anything about. It's not like anger where you can lose your temper and it comes bellowing out. Disgust is more of an internal ruminating that one often keeps to themselves and festers over time.

3. Grief

Grief can occur after a loss or through disaster and misfortune creating intense emotional suffering, acute sorrow and deep sadness. Grief is a universal reaction to bereavement. Furthermore, it can be feeling harassed, vexed or exasperated.

Grief comes in many forms and is something that we don't often "have time for." There are so many things humans have the tendency to grieve over. We often need to grieve over the loss of something we never attain (a job, for example), our expectations (the actions of a friend who doesn't meet them) and many many other things. It's easily overlooked because we don't see things as important enough to take the time to say "we're really feeling that loss," unless it's something we think is big enough like the death of a loved one.

4. Self-abuse

Abusing the self emotionally includes negative self-talk (e.g. "I'm such an idiot" 'I hate myself' 'I am ugly'), blaming the self, etc. Abusing the self physically includes mistreating the body by use of addictive substances; to not care for the body by lack of sleep, proper diet or nutrition; to work beyond what one can or should endure; to punish or tax oneself excessively. Illnesses can be forms of self-abuse (e.g. "I don't deserve to be healed.")

We are masters at this! This one becomes easily trapped because we do it so often and we are usually the last people we will give a break to. Many people are willing to forgive others more easily than themselves. In addition, many people think this is a helpful behaviour/emotion because it keeps them motivated and so on.

5. Unsupported

A lack of support, help or encouragement; not provided for by another; not defended when help is needed; feeling the burden is too heavy to bear alone.

This one goes back to being isolated. Feeling unsupported is scary and makes us feel like we have nowhere to turn. When we have nowhere to turn, we don't know what to do. And when that happens, we usually find a distraction and don't really work through the feelings and let them go.

6. Humiliation

A painful loss of pride, dignity or self-respect; to feel mortified; embarrassed.

This one comes up a lot! This is a very difficult thing to process because it's hard to admit and share our humiliation. Also, with society's expectations and how we tend to buy into them, we have plenty of opportunities to allow ourselves to feel humiliated over human mistakes, actions or simply how we look/act compared to what we think is the norm.

If you just learn one thing from this book, then it's been worth writing. I believe knowledge is power and with power comes great responsibility - now where have I heard that line before?

7. Overwhelm

To be overpowered in mind or emotion; extreme stress; feeling overpowered with superior force; feeling excessively burdened.

This is often self-inflicted. We live in a society where we never feel we're doing enough, fast enough, good enough. So, we take on more. And then we get overwhelmed. Also, we can tend to be overwhelmed with emotion and if we don't want to feel that, we can bury it and it can become trapped.

8. Worthless

Of no importance or value; without excellence of character, quality or esteem; serving no purpose.

So many of us have given other people permission to define our worth. We are so caught in a pattern of this that we just hang on to how we didn't live up to someone's expectations, or that they thought "x, y or z" about us. We hold tight to those perceptions, a part of our conditioning from childhood and are scared to let go of them, sometimes because we don't really know who we are; and sometimes because other people's perceptions of us serve us (let us "off the hook" for things we don't want to do, for example).

9. Lost

Unable to see the correct or acceptable course; having no direction. Physically lost most often shows up from childhood (e.g. being lost in the woods and can't find the way home). Emotionally lost refers to a feeling of being unable to see what the right decision or direction is; being unable to find emotional stability.

Feeling lost in life is so common. And, such a scary feeling. But, we often don't know how to get out of it. We don't take the time to really search for where we want to go next. It's often too scary to live our own truth and follow our dreams. We may be "at a loss" as to how to handle something as well. Being physically lost plays into being isolated and whenever we are alone during something scary, it tends to get trapped more easily; especially if we have no coping skills and no one to lean on to help us.

10. Conflict

Internal Conflict is a mental and emotional struggle within one's self, arising from opposing demands or impulses. (e.g. He was feeling conflicted about whether or not to take the new job). External Conflict is to fight; to disagree or be disagreeable; to struggle or battle against; to antagonise. Prolonged strife or struggle (e.g. She and her ex-husband experience continual conflict about custody of their children).

Conflict with others often gets stuck because we are programmed not to speak our truth; to not "rock the boat." This can be a real downfall because we can have a conflict with another person, but never push for an understanding and/or resolution of it, either of which would allow us to let it go. Far more common to be trapped in the body though, is an internal conflict. This is something we just couldn't follow our heart on, something we knew wasn't right but did anyway, or a time where one direction would make things easy but the other direction would make things harder for someone else or ourselves (you were internally conflicted). Often an internal conflict gets trapped because we did nothing at all; we decided to let life or someone else decide for us.

Now is the time, it's never too late, to take action, take responsibility, take your inner child by the hand, take time to tell you, you really care, share every moment together. Learning to love yourself is truly the greatest love of all and the key to becoming pain free.

''So keep your head high, keep your chin up, and most importantly, keep smiling, because life's a beautiful thing and there's so much to smile about.''

Marilyn Monroe

"There are only two ways to live your life. One is as though nothing is a miracle. The other is as though everything is a miracle."

Albert Einstein

'Secret to happiness, always have the mind of an adult, but the heart of a child'

Alexander Kupse

REFERENCES

BOOKS & WEBSITES YOU MAY LIKE TO TRY

'Sane New World' **Ruby Wax**

'Mind Over Medicine' **Lissa Rankin M.D**

'Letting Go The Pathway of Surrender' **David R. Hawkins M.D**

'The Alkaline Cure' **Dr Stephan Domenig**

Jason Vale Juice Master – **www.juicemaster.com**

'The Sugar Detox' **Brooke Alpert & Patricia Farris**

'You are what you Eat' **Gillian McKeith**

'Fat around the Middle' **Dr Marilyn Grenville**

www.fatbustforever.com, **Fiona Kirk** Nutritionist

'Rebound Exercise: The Ultimate Exercise for the New Millennium' **Albert E. Carter**

Information on PCD can be found on the UK website **www.pcdsupport.org.uk**

12125395R00076

Printed in Great Britain
by Amazon.co.uk, Ltd.,
Marston Gate.